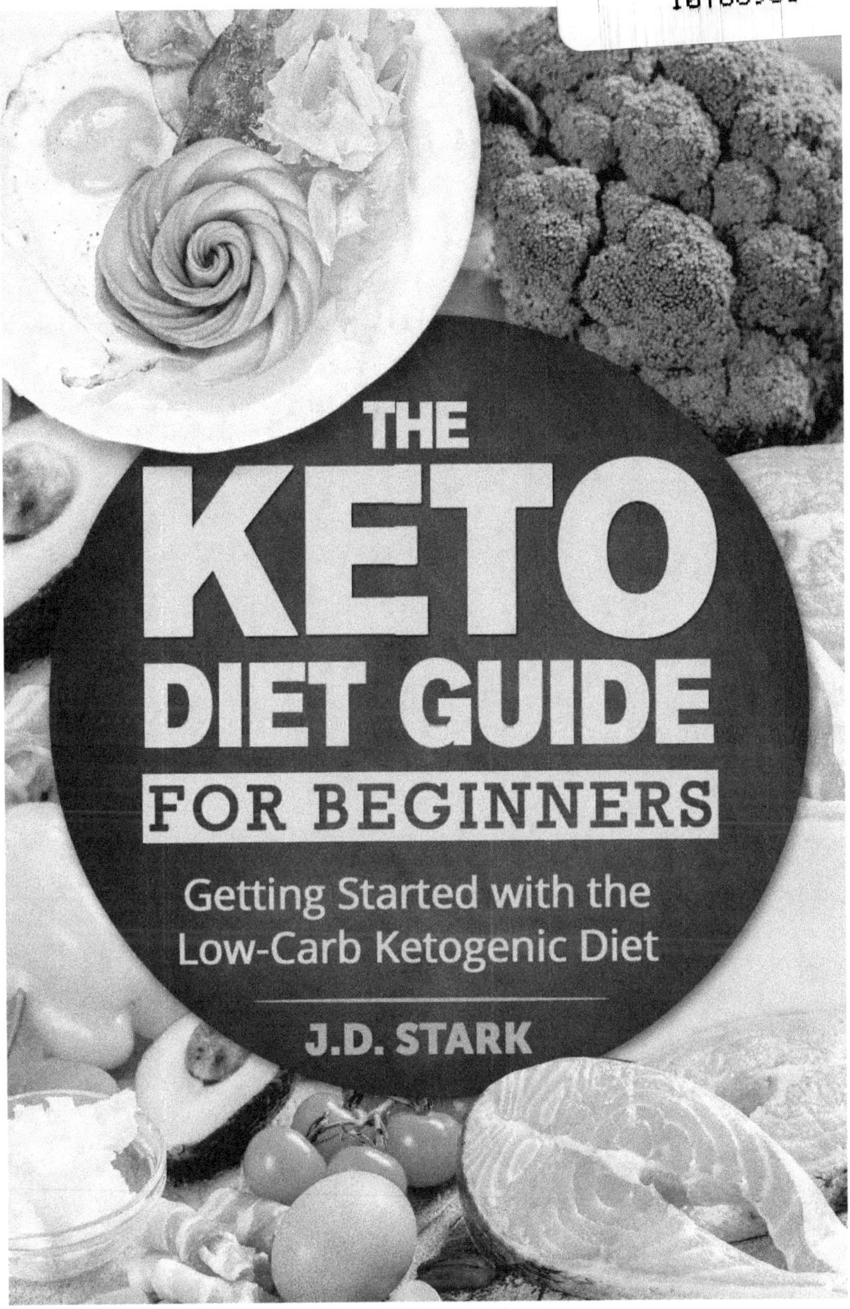

THE KETO DIET GUIDE

FOR BEGINNERS

Getting Started with the
Low-Carb Ketogenic Diet

J.D. STARK

The Keto Diet Guide for Beginners

Getting Started with the Low-Carb Ketogenic Diet

By J.D. Stark
jd-stark.com

Table of Contents

interim quality. Trademarks that mentioned are done without written consent and can in no way be considered an endorsement from the trademark holder.

Introduction

Congratulations on downloading your copy of The Keto Diet
Guide for Beginners: Getting Started with the Low-Carb Ketogenic
Diet. Thank you for doing so. Before you begin, take a moment to
understand the history of the ketogenic diet plan better.

History of the Keto Miracle
In 1924, Dr. Russell Wilder from the Mayo Clinic designed the
keto plan which was used as part of an epilepsy therapy treatment
plan since he also suffered from epilepsy. The plan became known
for its other effects which helped in weight loss and many other
ailments.

The program for ketosis was set aside in the 1940s because newer
methods were invented for the treatment of epilepsy. However,
during that time, 20-30% of the cases using the alternate plan had
failed. Therefore, the ketogenic plan was reintroduced to the
patients. As of 2016, Wilder is still functioning successfully
without the seizure episodes. It is also noted that the plan is
especially recommended for children.

As you begin your journey through the keto world, you will come
across many terms or abbreviations that you might not recognize.
Some of the simpler ones include (tbsp.) for tablespoon, (t) for
teaspoon, and (c.) for a cup.

These are a few more that you may see:
- Artificial Sweetener (AS) provides a zero/reduced carb
  count
- Extra-virgin olive oil (EVOO)
- Heavy Whipping Cream (HWC) is used by many cooks.
- Low-Carb and High-Fat (LCHF)
- Sugar-Free (SF)

You will be using extra-virgin olive oil (EVOO) for many of the recipes. You can make your own spray for using the olive oil spray by adding the oil to a spray bottle. You can also use canola oil which is another good choice for baking.

As time passes, you will become familiar with where each recipe is located, but for now, an index is offered after the conclusion of The Keto Diet Guide for Beginners: Getting Started with the Low-Carb Ketogenic Diet.

There are plenty of books focused on the ketogenic diet on the market, thanks again for choosing this one! Every effort was made to ensure it is full of as much useful information as possible. Please enjoy every tempting recipe.

Chapter 1: The Ketogenic Diet Plan

Flexibility or strictness is the name of the dieting game. Depending on your circumstances, you may not have the same goals as another individual. These are the three plans, so you are aware of the different levels:

Keto Method 1: The standard ketogenic diet (SKD) consists of high-fat, moderate protein, and is low in carbs.

Keto Method 2: The targeted keto diet, which is also called TKD, will provide you with a technique to add carbs to the diet plan during the times when you are working out.

Keto Method 3: The cyclical ketogenic diet or CKD is observed with five keto days followed by two high-carbohydrate days.

Keto Method 4: The high-protein keto diet is comparable to the standard keto plan (SKD) in all aspects. However, it does have more protein.

For now, as a beginner, you will be using the first method.

How the Keto Plan Works

A ketogenic diet will help you reduce your calorie intake to below the volume of calories your body can consume in one day. Therefore, you need to summon the energy which is stored in your fat cells to deliver fuel/energy to your muscles.

The keto diet will limit the volume of carbs you consume. A substantial portion of your daily fuel will come from fat content which is converted to ketones. A noticeable amount of fat burning is achieved with higher calories, and by sustaining food options used with the ketogenic plan. When you have the protein, carbohydrates, and fat ratio monitored by the diet plan such as the one shown in this cookbook; you are well on your way to a successful diet strategy.

You will not be over-eating with large portions of protein. You won't eliminate fat or carbs which makes it a useful and safe diet plan for fat loss. If you take the approach of eating less without considering your diet—you will be losing essential minerals and vitamins you need daily—which can result in muscle spasms, fatigue, mental fogginess, hunger, headaches, irritability, insomnia, and emotional depression. You can also lose valuable muscle mass; not just the pounds you intended to drop.

By using the lower carb keto plan, you can reduce your carbohydrates, calorie counts, and nurture your body with the suitable amount of water, meat, eggs, fish, veggies, and nuts, as well as high-quality oils which create fat loss minus the unpleasant side effects.

The Process
Ketosis is used to help you drop extra pounds and burn body fat using healthy eating practices. Proteins will fuel your body to burn the fat; which in turn, ketosis will maintain your muscles and make you less hungry.

Your body will remain healthy and work as it should. If you don't consume enough carbs from your food; your cells will begin to burn fat for the necessary energy instead. Your body will switch over to ketosis for its energy source as you cut back on your calories and carbs.

Elements of Ketosis: Lipogenesis & Glycogenesis

Two elements that occur when your body doesn't need the glucose:

- The Stage of Lipogenesis: If there is a sufficient supply of glycogen in your liver and muscles, any excess is converted to fat and stored.

- The Stage of Glycogenesis: The excess of glucose converts to glycogen and is stored in the muscles and liver. Research indicates that only about half of your energy used daily can be saved as glycogen.

When the glycerol and fatty acid molecules are released, the ketogenesis process begins, and acetoacetate is produced. The acetoacetate is converted to two types of ketone units:

- Acetone: This is mostly excreted as waste but can also be metabolized into glucose. This is the reason individuals on a ketogenic diet will experience a distinctive smelly breath.

- Beta-hydroxybutyrate or BHB: Your muscles will convert the acetoacetate into BHB which will fuel your brain after you have been on the keto diet for a short time.

Your body will have no more food (similar to when you are sleeping), making your body burn the fat to create ketones. Once the ketones break down the fats, which generate fatty acids, they will burn off in the liver through beta-oxidation.

Thus, when you no longer have a supply of glycogen or glucose, ketosis begins and will use the consumed/stored fat as energy. The Internet provides you with a keto calculator at "ketodietapp.com/Blog/page/KetoDiet-Buddy."

You can check your levels when you want to know what essentials your body needs during the course of your dieting plan or afterward. You will document your personal information such as height and weight. The calculator will provide you with the essential math.

For example, a 65-year old female – 176 lbs. – 5'1" with a sedentary lifestyle is calculated as 25% body fat. The calculator estimated the woman to consume 25 net carbs daily. This is the typical range to start the program (described below).

The Role of Calories, Protein, and Carbs

Carbs Needed Daily to Lose Weight

To achieve weight loss, you will need to reduce your carbohydrate intake. You will soon realize the plan will allow you to feel full and satisfied while still losing weight. You simply restrict carb intake including starches such as bread and pasta as well as sugars. As a result of the keto diet, you will replace them with fat and protein.

Not only will you lose weight; you will also lower blood pressure, triglycerides, and blood sugar.

What works for one person as a 'low-carb' diet, may be too low for another person. It depends on your activity levels, age, body composition, and gender. It may also depend on your metabolic health, food culture, and personal preferences. If you are more active and have more muscle mass; you can tolerate more carbs versus someone who is sedentary.

If people get the metabolic syndrome, he/she may become obese or suffer from type II diabetes whereas the rules change. It is sometimes referred to by the scientists as 'carbohydrate intolerance.'

As mentioned, there's no set rule for carb intake. These are some of the basic guidelines to consider as you blaze the path on the ketogenic diet plan, which is effective about 90% of the time:

Moderate Carb Intake: 100-150 Grams Daily
If you are active and lean, trying to maintain weight, these are some of the foods to consider:

- Several fruits daily
- All the veggies you can eat
- Healthy starches such as rice, oats, sweet potatoes, and potatoes

50-100 Grams Daily:
- Plenty of veggies
- 2-3 pieces of fruit each day
- Minimal intake of starchy carbs

20-50 Grams Daily:
Losing weight quickly falls into this category. If you have diabetes, are obese, or metabolically deranged, this is the plan for you. Consuming less than the 50 grams daily; your body will achieve a ketosis state which supplies the 'ketone bodies.'

Consider these guidelines:
- Some berries with whipped cream
- Plenty of low-carbohydrate veggies
- Trace carbs from foods including nuts, seeds, and avocados

As you now see, it is important to experiment and categorize where you fall on the scales before you make any changes. Seek your doctor's advice before changing your eating patterns. In some cases, you could reduce the need for some medications.

The 5-Steps to Achieve Ketosis

Step 1: Lower Your Carb Consumption

The most important element in achieving ketosis is a very low-carbohydrate diet. Your cells normally use the sugar/glucose as the main fuel source, but most of your cells can also use other sources for fuel such as fatty acids as well as ketones.

When the carb intake is lowered, the levels of the insulin hormone decline which allows the fatty acids to be released from fat storage in your body.

Some individuals need to limit their intake of net carbs. To discover the net carbs in a recipe, you will take the total of the carbs minus (-) the fiber content or up to 20 grams each day. Whereas, others can remain in ketosis while eating twice that amount. If you can restrict your consumption to less than 20 grams for the first 2 weeks, you will be certain that ketosis is reached. At that time, you can relax and maintain the ketosis state.

Step 2: Increase the Healthy Fat Intake to Your Ketogenic Diet Plan

Forget the old sayings of it has too much fat. Consuming plenty of healthy fats can help boost your ketone levels. The lowered carbohydrate intake teams up with the high fats to produce ketosis. If you are using the ketogenic diet for weight loss, you can also achieve 60-80% of your calories from fat. Note, the typical diet plan for epilepsy is higher with 85-90% of the calories from fat.

It is important to use high-quality food sources since you are consuming such a large percentage of your diet from fat intake. Consider using these good fats for your cooking needs; butter, coconut oil, avocado oil, tallow, and lard. You will soon discover how many high-fat foods are low in carbs, but you still need to count them to prevent losing the ketosis state. In general, you should consume a minimum of 60% of calories from fat to boost the ketone levels. Choose from both animal and plant sources.

Step 3: Incorporate Coconut Oil into Your Keto Diet Plan

The oil is also used as one of the best ways to improve ketone levels in people with nervous system disorders, such as those with Alzheimer's disease.

Medium-chain triglycerides (MCTs) are contained in coconut oil which speeds up the ketosis process. Unlike many other fats, the MCTs are absorbed rapidly and go straight to your liver where they are consumed for immediate energy – resulting in conversion to ketones. The oil contains four types of these fats, 50% of which comes from lauric acid.

Research has indicated the higher percentage may produce sustained ketosis levels because it is metabolized more gradual than other MCTs. Add coconut oil slowly to your diet because it can cause some stomach cramping or diarrhea until you adjust. Begin with 1 t. each day. Increase the amount up to 2-3 tbsp. over the span of a week.

Step 4: Maintain Protein Intake

You must supply your liver with amino acids which can be used for making new glucose (gluconeogenesis). Your liver produces the glucose for the cells and organs in your body that cannot use ketones as fuel. This includes portions of the brain, kidneys, and red blood cells.

Protein also maintains muscle mass when the carb intake is lowered, especially during a weight loss program. Research has indicated your physical performance, and the preservation of your muscle mass is at maximum speed when your intake range is 0.55-0.77 grams per pound of lean mass.

Think of it in simple terms. Excessive protein intake may suppress ketone production, whereas consuming too little can lead to muscle mass loss.

Step 5: Test the Ketone Levels & Adjust the Diet Plan

Maintaining ketosis is an individual process, and you need to be sure you are achieving your goals. The levels of acetone, acetoacetate, and beta-hydroxybutyrate can be measured in your breath, urine, and blood.
You can use a Ketonix which is a meter to measure your breath. You breathe into the meter, and a specific color will flash to indicate your levels of ketosis.

You can also measure the ketones with a blood ketone meter which works similar to a glucose meter. Add a small drop of blood on a testing strip and insert the tab into the meter. It will indicate the amount of beta-hydroxybutyrate in your bloodstream. This process has been researched as a valid indicator of the current ketosis levels. Unfortunately, the strips are expensive.

Thirdly, test your urine for acetoacetates. The strip is dipped into the urine which will change the color of the strip. The various shades of purple and pink indicate the levels of the ketones. The darker the color on the testing strip; the higher the level of ketones. The major benefit is they are inexpensive. The most effective time to test is early in the morning - after a ketogenic diet dinner the evening before testing.

You should use one or more of these methods to indicate whether you need to adjust your intake of foods to remain in ketosis.

How Long Before Ketosis

When you fast, the hormones in your body will change. The keto plan is similar to this process. You could achieve ketosis in just a couple of days once you have used up all of your stored glycogen. It can take a month, a week, or just a few days. It all depends on which type of method you choose (previously explained). Your protein and carbohydrate intake will determine the time. Exercise also plays a vital role.

How to Know When You Are in Ketosis
Whether you have taken any tests to discover your ketosis status, your body will exhibit physical signs to prompt you. You may have a loss of appetite, increased thirst, have bad breath, or notice a stronger urine smell. These are all clues from your body.

Ketosis and Your Sleep Patterns
After you have a good night of sleep, your body is in ketosis since you have fasted for over eight hours, and you are on the way to burning ketones. If you are new to the high-fat and low-carb dieting, the optimal fat-burning state takes time. Your body has depended on bringing in carbs and glucose; it will not readily give up carbs and start to crave saturated fats.
A restless night is also a normal side effect. Vitamin supplements can sometimes remedy the problem that can be caused by a lowered insulin and serotonin level. For a quick fix; try one-half of a tablespoon of fruit spread and a square of chocolate. It sounds crazy, but it works!

Lowered Appetite
When you reduce your carbs and proteins, you will be increasing your fat intake. The reduced appetite comes from the multitude of fibrous veggies, fats, and satiating nutrients provided in the new diet.

The full-factor is a huge benefit to the ketogenic plan. It will give you one less thing to worry about – being hungry.

Thirst is Increased
Fluid retention is increased when you are consuming carbohydrates. Once the carbs are flushed away, water weight is lost. You counter-balance by increasing the water intake since you are probably dehydrated.

The ketogenic diet requires more water since as a result, you are storing carbs. If you are dehydrated; your body can use the stored carbs to restore hydration. When you're in ketosis, the carbs are removed, and your body doesn't have the water reserves. If you have tried other diets, you might have been dehydrated, but the higher carbohydrate counts stopped you from being thirsty. Thus, the keto state is a diuretic state, so drink plenty of water daily.

Bad Breath Flares
You may notice a metallic or fruity taste with an odor similar to nail polish remover. This is the by-product of acetoacetic acid (acetone) which is an obvious indication of ketosis. You may also experience a drier mouth. These changes are normal as a side effect as your body processes these high-fat foods.

Once you are accustomed to the ketogenic dieting techniques, the bad breath symptoms will pass. If you are socializing, try a diet soda or a non-sugary drink. Sugar-free gum is also a quick fix. Always check the nutrition labels for carbohydrate facts; you may be surprised. Diet soda and gum is not generally allowed on the keto diet because they reduce ketones. Therefore, only use it temporarily. If you are at home, just grab the toothbrush.

Pungent Urine Smells
With the high acetone levels, your urine is also a strong clue to ketosis. There is no reason for concern; it's just your body adjusting to the new status.

Digestive Issues
You have made a huge change in your diet overnight; it's expected you may have problems including constipation or diarrhea when you first start the keto diet. Each person is different, and it will depend on what foods you have chosen to eat to increase your fiber intake using various vegetables.

You may experience issues because your fiber intake may be too high in comparison to your previous diet. Try reducing new foods until the transitional phase of ketosis is concluded. It should clear up with time.

You may be lacking beneficial bacteria. Try consuming fermented foods to increase your probiotics and aid digestion. You can benefit from B vitamins, omega 3 fatty acids, and beneficial enzymes as well.

Other Possible Side Effects
Heart Palpitations
You may begin to feel 'fluttery' as a result of dehydration or because of an insufficient intake of salt. Try to make adjustments, but if you don't feel better quickly, you should seek emergency care.

Induction Flu
The diet can make you irritable, nauseous, a bit confused, lethargic, and possibly suffer from a headache. Several days into the plan should remedy these effects. If not, add one-half of a teaspoon of salt to a glass of water, and drink it to help with the side effects. You may need to do this once a day for about the first week, and it could take about 15 to 20 minutes before it helps. It will go away!

Leg Cramps
The loss of magnesium (a mineral) can be a demon and create a bit of pain with the onset of the keto diet plan changes. With the loss of the minerals during urination, you could experience bouts of cramps in your legs.

Constipation
During the ketogenic plan, you must drink plenty of water of you could easily become constipated because of dehydration. The low-carbs contribute to the issue. Eat the right veggies and add a small

amount of salt to your food to help with the movements. If all else fails, try some Milk of Magnesia.

Chapter 2: Create a Ketogenic Inventory

These are the steps you should take before you plunge into your new diet plan.
Stock Your Cabinets for the Keto Plan

You can prepare almost any meal if you have the right items readily available. By stocking the ingredients in the refrigerator, freezer, or cabinets; you can always stay on track. Begin with these items:

Dairy Products

It is important to maintain your health using dairy products. It is best to choose fresh/raw or organic milk products. You can also add additional protein and calcium using non-dairy products such as cashew or almond milk. Keep these in the fridge:

- Heavy cream
- Butter
- Cream cheese
- Sour cream
- Ghee
- Parmesan cheese
- Sharp cheddar cheese

Protein Products

The keto plan focuses on quality proteins. You can use many of these items listed as a starting point:

- Tuna: Fresh & canned
- Salmon: Fresh wild caught salmon – portion in bags to freeze
- Eggs
- Shrimp

- Fresh nuts: Macadamia, sesame seeds, flax seeds, chia seeds, etc.
- Turkey: Breasts & ground turkey
- Pork Chops
- Chicken: Thighs, breasts, drumsticks, & ground chicken
- Beef: Flank steak, chuck roast, sirloin, lean ground beef
- Venison: This is a good choice since it is lean and vegetarian raised meat.

Healthy Fats

To achieve success on the ketogenic diet, you need fats. These are some of those good fats:

- Avocado
- Extra-virgin olive oil (EVOO)
- Sesame, avocado, and coconut oil
- Flaxseed oil
- Coconut flakes
- Olives

Vegetables

Many of the vegetables have a lot of carbohydrates. You will want to consider these:

- Asparagus
- Broccoli
- Cauliflower
- Onions
- Bell pepper
- Cabbage
- Lettuce
- Tomatoes - limited
- Parsnips
- Radishes
- Bell Peppers

- Squash
- Peas
- Spinach
- Squash
- Turnip
- Zucchini

Pantry Items

These are some of the favorites to use while on the ketogenic diet:

- Coconut flour
- Quinoa
- Splenda & Stevia
- Sugar-free ketchup
- Sugar-free gelatin
- Unsweetened cocoa powder
- Yellow mustard
- Pickles (limit sweet or bread & butter)
- Natural nut butter – no sugar

Other Essential Foods for the Ketogenic Diet Plan

As you read through your Keto Crock Pot Cookbook, you will notice many of these items used frequently. Try to keep these in your well-stocked kitchen:

- Grass-Fed Butter: You can promote fat loss and is almost carb-free. The butter is a naturally occurring fatty acid which is rich in conjugated linoleic acid (CLA). It is good for maintaining weight loss and retaining lean muscle mass.

- Avocados: Purchase this healthy food which has 24 grams – 30 grams of healthy fats, and is also high in fiber.

- Eggs: Many quick meals can be prepared with the easy and versatile eggs.

- Kale: Your heart health can be greatly improved with the rich nutrients including magnesium and folate.

- Olives: You can use olives in many recipes and salads with its high fiber and fat counts.

- Coconut Oil: Your body quickly converts the MCTs within the oil into energy.

Your list will grow as you experiment with your new recipes.

7 Best Sweeteners for the Ketogenic Diet Plan

These sweeteners are listed from the most to least popular. Consider each one of these sweeteners before you make a choice. The recipes are usually flexible, but many typically recommend using a specific product.

Choice 1: The best all-around sweetener is Pyure's Organic All-Purpose Blend. There is not a bitter aftertaste with this stevia-based product. The blend of stevia and erythritol is an excellent alternative to sweetening, baking, and cooking needs. It is suggested that you substitute 1/3 teaspoon of Pyure for every one teaspoon of sugar. Adjust this to your taste, since you can always add a bit more.

For powdered sugar, you can grind the sweetener in a NutriBullet/blender until it's very dry.

Choice 2: The Swerve Granular Sweetener is also a superb choice as a blend made from non-digestible carbs sourced from starchy root veggies and select fruits. It is an excellent choice for those who do not like the taste of stevia.

Swerve is on the market as a one-to-one substitute. However, start with ¾ of a teaspoon for every one of sugar. Increase the portion as needed. Swerve also has its own confectioners/powdered sugar for your baking needs. On the downside, it is more expensive (about twice) than other products such as the Pyure. You have to decide if it's worth the difference.

Choice 3: The Purist is provided by NOW Foods has a 100% erythritol sweetener. The product is about 70% sweet as sugar. Therefore, you need a little more. Consider using 1 1/3 to 1 ½ teaspoons of the erythritol in comparison to one of sugar.

Choice 4: Xylitol has recently been added to the topside of the sugary list. It is excellent for sweetening your teriyaki and BBQ sauce, and it tastes just like sugar!
The natural occurring sugar alcohol has the Glycemic index (GI) standing of 13. If you have tried others, this might be for you. Some have reported a slightly minty aftertaste.

The xylitol is also known to keep your mouth bacteria in check and improving your dental health. It is commonly found in chewing gum. In large amounts, it can cause diarrhea - which gum can be considered as a laxative if used in large quantities.

Note: If you have a puppy in the house, be sure to use caution since it is toxic to dogs (even small amounts).

Choice 5: Sukrin Gold has a brown sugar alternative. The mixture of stevia and erythritol claims the one-to-one ratio for sugar. It is always best to start with the rate of ¾ of a teaspoon per one teaspoon of sugar. According to the standards in the United States, this is not a good choice if you are seeking a gluten-free alternative. It contains malt extract.

Choice 6: Stevia Drops are offered by Sweet Leaf and offer flavors including English toffee, hazelnut, vanilla, and chocolate. You can make a sweetened coffee and drinks quickly. However, everyone is different, and some believe the drops to be too bitter to taste. Only use three drops to equal one teaspoon of sugar.

Choice 7: Syrup choices are needed, especially for pancakes. You can choose Lakanto's Maple-flavored sugar-free syrup since it is monk-fruit and erythritol based. You can also select the Golden Monk Fruit Sweetener as a brown sugar choice. The name monk-fruit came from the Buddhist monks over 1,000 years ago. It is considered a cooling-agent and may not agree with your digestive system. Use it sparingly if using in baked goods.

Foods to Limit
You may use these sometimes, but try to limit the amounts used. Always count for the extra carbs in your recipes. These are a few of the ones to use occasionally- if you have a craving:

- Agave Nectar: One teaspoon has 5 grams of carbs versus 4 grams of table sugar.

- Beans and Legumes: This group to avoid includes peas, lentils, kidney beans, and chickpeas. If you use them; be sure to count the carbs, protein, and fat content.

- Cashews and Pistachios: The high carb content should be monitored for these yummy nuts.

- Fruits: Raspberries, blueberries, and cranberries contain a high sugar content. In small portions; you can enjoy some strawberries, apples, or pears.

- Hydrogenated Fats: Cold-pressed items should be avoided when using vegetable oils such as safflower, olive, soybean, or flax. Coronary heart disease has been linked to these fats which also include margarine.

- Potatoes and potato products

- Corn and corn products

- Alcohol Products: You need to limit the intake of your alcoholic drinks which will include:
    1. Beer
    2. Flavored liquor
    3. Cocktails
    4. Dry Wine
    5. Mixers: Soda, Juice, or Syrup

However, some of the professionals have discovered these might be acceptable:

- Rum: Choose the ones with zero carbs or sugar.
- Tequila: The agave plant is the source of tequila.
- Vodka: Check the carb content since it is usually produced (grain-based) from rye, potatoes, and wheat.
- Whiskey, Barley, corn, rye, and wheat are the grains used which have zero carbs or sugar.

Note: This doesn't promote you drinking alcohol, but it does produce ketones in the liver. Remember, it still needs to be consumed in small amounts to prevent any health issues.

You should also avoid sugar including these:
- Dextrose
- Corn syrup
- Fructose
- Honey Maltose
- Maple syrup

Supplements you can use to stay on the ketogenic diet

Fish Oil: Purchase this at any health food store in either the liquid or capsule form. The oil provides a natural anti-inflammatory content. It also contributes to the higher fat intake requirements on the ketogenic diet.

Creatine: This amino acid is favored by bodybuilders and athletes. It can be purchased either from a health food store or online with Amazon. Its most beneficial feature is for strengthening and building lean muscle mass as well as enhancing athletic performance.

MCT Oil: As mentioned coconut and palm oil are great ways to get your medium chain triglycerides level inline. You can also get it from yogurt and cheese. If you want a simpler method for whatever reason, try using MCT powder or oil in your cooking. It is well known for its long-lasting energy benefits, and high-fat content. You can purchase the oil from Amazon.
Perfect Keto: You can use this powdered drink supplement to help spike your ketone levels. Don't be mistaken; this cannot replace the keto diet plan. It is a good 'stand-by' if you exceed your carb limit. It can only assist to keep you in ketosis.

Chapter 3: Tips to Transition into the Ketogenic Diet

It is a challenging process when you make a choice to change to a low-carbohydrate lifestyle. It takes a lot of willpower to refuse some sugary treats your family and friends can consume and not gain an ounce of body fat. However, you will be ahead of the game plan by using some of these suggestions. The keto plan works, and you can use it whether you are at home or on-the-go. These are the guidelines:

- Journalize: Keep a journal of everything you eat. If you cheat, that has to count also. It will be a reminder of your indulgence, but it will help keep you on track. Others may believe you are obsessed with the plan, but it is your health and well-being that you are improving.

- Market Time: When you go to the supermarket, take your new skills, a grocery list, and read each of the labels for hiding carbs.

- Control the Kitchen: One of the easiest ways to stay on your plan is to remove the temptations. Remove the chocolate, candy, bread, pasta, rice, and sugary sodas you have supplied in your kitchen. If you live alone, this is an easy task. It is a bit more challenging if you have a family. The diet will also be useful for them if you plan your meals using some of the recipes included in this book.

- Count the Carbs: In today's society, almost every consumable product purchased has the nutrient labeling on the package. Check them before you take them home. It may take a bit of extra time when you plan a shopping adventure. It is essential to check the panels on every item to keep the ketosis in check. It might be a complicated process at first, but it is worth the effort.

Exercise to Meet Success

Short exercises of approximately 21 minutes daily have been scientifically proven to be more beneficial than longer workouts. For many years, trainers believed in sit-ups and push-ups with endless repetitions; but not today!

When you're working out on a treadmill or stationary bike; you're building up the cortisol in your body which is a stress hormone that helps burn fat. However, if you have a lot of exercises planned, your body will move into a protection mode. This mode will cause storage of fat around your midsection which can put you at risk for diabetes, heart disease, or possibly cancer.

The type of plan that will work for you is a high-intensity interval training (HIIT) technique. Work-out in short intervals any time of the day you feel the need to get moving. You just need fast feet, and high knee lifts to perform your exercises. After all, you are trying to push your heart to its maximum, not your biceps.

Cortisol Levels and Exercise

Firstly, you need to understand that cortisol is a hormone which is released from your adrenal gland in response to chemical signs or other stress signals. The release of cortisol in long workouts, such as jogging, and the adverse effects of the release of high doses of cortisol for weight loss are essential elements in your successful program. The hormone creates the fight-or-flight reaction as a result of the additional activity/stress during your workout.

Chapter 4: Benefits of the Keto Diet & the 7-Day Plan

The ketogenic diet is an excellent plan and aids in some of the following illnesses:

- Improved Thinking Skills: Your brain is approximately 60% fat by weight. Therefore, you might become confused as you consume high-fat foods. By increasing your fatty foods intake; you will have better chances to better your mind. It can maintain itself and work at full capacity.

- Obesity and Overweight Individuals: Many people exceed what is considered healthy figures when it comes to weight. It is imperative to use the keto diet plan to get started on the right path for weight loss.

- Acne: By eating fewer processed foods and less sugar; your insulin levels will be lowered, and any acne issues should improve.

- Alzheimer's Disease: The disease's progression can be slowed and the symptoms reduced by using the keto plan.

- Cancer: Several types of cancer and slow tumor growths are being treated using the keto diet.

- Prediabetes and Diabetes: Excess fat is removed with the keto plan, which is what is linked to pre-diabetes, type-2 diabetes, and metabolic syndrome. In one study, insulin sensitivity was improved by 75%. Similar results with type-2 diabetes patients indicated that out of 21 participants, seven were successful in eliminating all of the medications related to diabetes.

- Epilepsy: Reductions from seizures have occurred in children who use the ketogenic diet. The therapeutic keto diet used for epilepsy often restricts the carbs to less than 15 grams of carbs each day to further raise the ketone levels. Don't try this unless you have the supervision of a medical professional.

- Gum Disease and Tooth Decay: The pH balance in your mouth is influenced by sugar intake. Your gum issues could subside after about three months on a keto diet plan. You will be consuming healthier foods.

- Lower Blood Pressure: Low-carb diets are an excellent way to reduce your blood pressure. It is advisable to speak with your physician about lowering your meds while on the plan. If you begin to feel dizzy; that is one of the first signs the lack of carbs is working. You are headed in the right direction.

- Improvement of your Cholesterol Profile: An arterial buildup is generally associated with your triglyceride and cholesterol levels, which have been proven to improve with the keto diet plan.

- Joint Pain and Stiffness: Grain-based foods are eliminated from your diet on the keto plan. It is believed the grains can be one of the biggest causes of pain or chronic illness. After all, it has been said before, "no pain –no grain."

- Lack of Hunger: This vast benefit happens because fat is naturally more satisfying than just carbs. You just need to wait a little longer to become satiated after a meal. The high-carbs will cause the full-state to last longer.

Meal Plan – 7 Days
The following meal plan is a general outline for you as you learn
how easy it is to remain on a ketogenic diet plan. With the
calculations provided, you can easily enjoy a few extras, if you
count those carbs.
Enjoy every meal with no worries!

7-Day Keto Plan

Monday:
Breakfast: Cream Cheese Scrambled Eggs - Net Carbs: 1.3 g
Lunch: Pesto Turkey Meatballs – Net Carbs: 0.5 g
Dinner: Rib Eye Steak Salad – Net Carbs: 1.5 g
Snacks: Sesame Sugar Candied Pecans - Net Carbs: 4 g

Tuesday:
Breakfast: Key Lime Pie Smoothie - Net Carbs: 2 g
Lunch: Stuffed Pork Tenderloin – Net Carbs: 2.9 g
Dinner: Sesame Ginger Salmon – Net Carbs: 2.5 g
            With Bacon & Cabbage Net Carbs: 7 g
Dessert: No-Bake Cheesecake - Net Carbs: 5 g

Wednesday:
Breakfast: Maple Pumpkin Flaxseed Muffins – Net Carbs: 2 g
Lunch: Parmesan Chicken – Net Carbs: 6 g
Dinner: Steak with Mushroom Port Sauce – Net Carbs: 6 g
            With Roasted Radishes – 2 g.
Dessert: Blueberry Cream Pie - Net Carbs: 3 g

Thursday:
Breakfast: Stuffed Avocado with Egg Salad – Net Carbs: 3.03 g
Lunch: Chicken Breast Salad with Vinaigrette Pressurized – Net
Carbs: 11 g
Dinner: Cheeseburger Calzone – Net Carbs: 3 g
            With Zucchini Fries – Net Carbs: 4.5 g
Snacks or Dessert: Chocolate Chip Cookies - Net Carbs: 2 g

Friday:
Breakfast: Blueberry Pancakes – Net Carbs: 5.78 g
Lunch: Bacon Chicken Ranch Casserole – Net Carbs: 2 g
Dinner: Cod in the Skillet – Net Carbs – 1 g
            With Brussels Sprouts – Net Carbs: 6.8 g
Snack or Dessert: Avocado Mint Green Smoothie - Net Carbs: 5 g

Saturday:
Breakfast: Roasted Mushroom & Cauliflower Grits- Net Carbs: 11.28 g
Lunch: Bacon Wrapped Scallops – Net Carbs: 3 g
Dinner: Balsamic Beef Pot Roast – Net Carbs: 3 g
Dessert or Snack: Mocha 5-Minute Smoothie - Net Carbs: 4 g

Sunday:
Breakfast: Blueberry Yogurt Smoothie - Net Carbs: 2 g
Lunch: Zesty Shrimp – Net Carbs – 2.5 g
Dinner: Beef Wellington – Net Carbs: 2.31 g
            With Spaghetti Squash & Cheese – Net Carbs: 4.8 g
Snacks or Dessert: Coconut Macaroons Fat Bombs - Net Carbs: 0.5 g

How easy is that? You still have plenty of carbs allowed for you to do as you choose. All you need to do is follow the given guidelines for snacks, and you will be well on the way to maintaining your ketosis state of being. You can always use the leftovers!

Chapter 5: Keto Breakfast in Style

No matter what you're craving, it starts with a great breakfast plan!

Cream Cheese Scrambled Eggs

Ingredients
2 eggs
1 tbsp. whipping cream
2 t. butter
2 tbsp. cream cheese
Pepper and salt

Instructions
1. Whisk the eggs, salt, pepper, and whipping cream.
2. Heat a saucepan and melt the butter. Empty the egg mixture and diced-up cream cheese to the pan. Stir gently and continue until the eggs are done.
3. Give it a sprinkle of salt and pepper. Serve and enjoy!

Servings: 2
Calories: 180.8 | Protein: 7.9 g | Net Carbs: 1.3 g | Fat: 15.9 g

Roasted Mushroom & Cauliflower Grits

Ingredients
6 oz. sliced baby Portobello mushrooms
1 tbsp. rosemary
3 minced garlic cloves
½ c. chopped walnuts
2 tbsp. olive oil
½ c. water
1 med. cauliflower
1 c. of each:
    -Half & Half
    -Shredded sharp cheddar cheese

To Taste: Salt
2 tbsp. butter

Instructions
1. Warm up the oven to 400°F. Cover a baking tin with aluminum foil.
2. In a small container, mix the smoked paprika, rosemary, walnuts, mushrooms, and garlic. Coat the mixture with the oil, and sprinkle with the salt.
3. Spread the mixture into the prepared pan and roast 15 minutes.
4. Pulse the cauliflower in the processor until fine.
5. In a medium pot, boil ½ cup of water and add the grits-cauliflower.
6. Pour in the Half & Half, and simmer about three minutes on the med-low setting on the stovetop. Slowly add in ¼ cup of water if you like your grits thinner until you have them the way you want them.
7. Mix in the butter and cheese – heating until well combined and creamy. Sprinkle with salt as desired. When the mushrooms have browned, use them to top off the bowl of hot grits and enjoy.

Servings: 4
Calories: 455 | Protein: 15.28 g | Net Carbs: 11.28 g | Fat: 36.5 g

Stuffed Avocado with Egg Salad

Ingredients
1/3 med. red onion
6 large hard-boiled eggs
3 celery ribs
4 tbsp. mayonnaise
2 tbsp. fresh lime juice
2 t. brown mustard
Pepper & salt to taste

½ t. cumin
1 t. hot sauce
3 med. avocados

Instructions
1. Begin by chopping the onions, celery, and eggs. Combine with all of the other fixings except for the avocado.
2. Slice the avocado and remove the pit. Scoop the salad into the avocado and serve!

Servings: 6
Calories: 280.57 | Protein: 8.32 g | Net Carbs: 3.03 g | Fat: 24.83 g

On the Sweeter Side

Blueberry Pancakes

Ingredients
¾ c. ricotta
3 large eggs
¼ c. unsweetened vanilla almond milk
½ t. vanilla extract
1 c. almond flour
¼ t. salt
½ c. golden flaxseed meal
¼ - ½ t. stevia powder
1 t. baking powder
¼ c. blueberries

Instructions
1. Prepare a skillet over the medium heat setting. Combine the ricotta, eggs, milk, and vanilla extract. Blend the stevia, baking powder, flour, salt, and flaxseed meal in another dish.

2. Add the dry with the wet ingredients into a blender, slowly, until a batter forms. For each ¼ cup of batter; add two to three blueberries.
3. Add butter to the skillet. When it melts, pour the batter in and brown. Flip when browned.
4. Serve with additional berries or a drizzle of sugar-free syrup.

Servings: 5
Calories: 311.4| Protein: 15.25 g | Net Carbs: 5.78 g | Fat: 22.61 g

Maple Pumpkin Flaxseed Muffins

Ingredients
1 ¼ c. ground flaxseeds
½ tbsp. baking powder
1/3 c. erythritol
1 tbsp. of each:
    -Cinnamon
    -Pumpkin pie spice
½ t. salt
2 tbsp. coconut oil
1 c. pure pumpkin puree
1 egg
½ t. of each:
    -Vanilla extract
    -Apple cider vinegar
¼ c. maple syrup
Useful Appliances: Blender such as NutriBullet
Garnish: Pumpkin seeds

Instructions
    1. Set the oven temperature to 350ºF.
    2. Prepare a muffin tin large enough for ten muffins with silicone cupcake liners or grease the tin.

3. Add the seeds to the blender about one second – no longer or it could become damp.
4. Combine the dry fixings and whisk until well mixed. Add the puree, vanilla extract, and pumpkin spice. Add the maple syrup (1/2 t.) if using.
5. Blend in the oil, egg, and apple cider vinegar. Combine nuts or any other add-ins of your choice.
6. Scoop the mixture out by the tablespoon into the prepared tins. Garnish with some of the pumpkin seeds. Leave a little space in the top, since they will rise.
7. Bake approximately 20 minutes. They are ready when they are slightly browned. Let them cool a few minutes and add some ghee/butter or some more syrup.

Servings: 10
Calories: 120 | Fat: 8.5 g | Net Carbs: 2 g | Protein: 5 g

Delicious Smoothies

These healthy drinks are fantastic for breakfast or a snack. Enjoy each one!

Avocado Mint Green Smoothie

Ingredients
½ c. almond milk
¾ c. full-fat coconut milk
½ avocado (3-4 oz.)
3 sprigs cilantro
5-6 large mint leaves
¼ t. vanilla extract
1 squeeze - lime juice
Sweetener of your choice – to taste
1 ½ c. crushed ice

Instructions
1. Measure each of the fixings and add to the blender.
2. Combine using the low-speed setting until pureed.
3. Toss in the ice and mix. Serve in a chilled glass.

Servings: 1
Calories: 223 | Protein: 1 g |Fats: 23 g | Net Carbs: 5 g

Blueberry – Banana Smoothie

Ingredients
1 tbsp. chia seeds
3 tbsp. golden flaxseed meal
2 c. vanilla unsweetened coconut milk
¼ c. blueberries
10 drops liquid stevia
2 tbsp. MCT oil
¼ t. xanthan gum
1 ½ t. banana extract

Instructions

1. Pour the milk and add the flaxseed meal, chia seeds, blueberries, MCT oil, liquid stevia, xanthan gum, and banana extract.
2. Blend for one to two minutes until all of the fixings are well mixed.
3. Serve with some ice (before or after mixing) in a couple of cold glasses.

Servings: 2
Calories: 264 |Fats: 25 g | Protein: 4 g | Net Carbs: 3 g

Blueberry Yogurt Smoothie

Ingredients
10 blueberries
½ c. yogurt
½ t. vanilla extract
1 c. coconut milk
Stevia to taste

Instructions

1. Add all of the fixings into the blender, mixing well.
2. When creamy, pour into 2 chilled mugs and enjoy.

Servings: 2
Calories: 70 | Protein: 2 g |Fats: 5 g | Net Carbs: 2 g

Key Lime Pie Smoothie

Ingredients
½ avocado
1 c. coconut milk
2 limes – juiced and zest
Sweetener of your choice – to taste
1 cup of ice

Instructions
1. Toss in the avocado along with the zest and juice of a lime, sweetener, milk, and the ice.
2. Blend until smooth and serve in a couple of frosty glasses.

Servings: 2
Calories: 88 | Protein: 1 g |Fats: 8 g | Net Carbs: 2 g

Mocha 5-Minute Smoothie

Ingredients
1 ½ c. unsweetened almond milk
½ c. coconut milk – from the can
2 t. instant coffee crystals – regular or decaffeinated
1 t. vanilla extract
3 tbsp. of each:
    -Erythritol blend/granulated stevia
    -Unsweetened cocoa powder
1 avocado

Instructions
1. Slice the avocado into halves. Discard the pit and scoop out the center. Add it along with the rest of the ingredients into the blender.
2. Mix until smooth and serve.

Servings: 3
Calories: 176 | Protein: 3 g |Fats: 16 g | Net Carbs: 4 g

Beef Dishes
Balsamic Beef Pot Roast
Ingredients
1 boneless (approx. 3 lb.) chuck roast
1 t. of each:
    -Garlic powder
    -Black ground pepper
1 tbsp. kosher salt
¼ c. balsamic vinegar
½ c. chopped onion
2 c. water
¼ t. xanthan gum
For the Garnish: Freshly chopped parsley

Instructions
1. Combine the garlic powder, salt, and pepper and rub the chuck roast with the mixture.
2. Use a heavy skillet to sear the roast. Add the vinegar and deglaze the pan as you continue cooking for one more minute.
3. Toss the onion to a pot of the (two cups) boiling water along with the roast. Cover with a top and simmer for three to four hours on a low setting.
4. Take the meat from the pot and add to a cutting surface. Shred into chunks and remove any fat or bones.
5. Add the xanthan gum to the broth and whisk. Place the roast meat back in the pan to warm up.
6. Serve with a favorite side dish.

Servings: 10
Calories: 393| Protein: 30 g | Net Carbs: 3 g | Fat: 28 g

Beef Wellington
Ingredients

2 (4 lb.) tenderloin steaks
Salt and pepper to taste
1 tbsp. butter
½ c. almond flour
1 c. shredded mozzarella cheese
4 tbsp. liver pate

Instructions
1. Program the oven temperature to 400°F.
2. Pepper and salt the steaks and melt the butter on the med-high heat setting on the stovetop. Arrange the meat in the pan when it's hot and sear on all sides. Flip them over every two or three minutes. Let it cool.
3. Heat up the cheese in a microwave about one minute. Stir in the flour to form a dough. Use a rolling pin and place the dough in between two pieces of parchment paper to flatten it. Create a round ball.
4. Add one tablespoon of the pate into the dough, large enough to fit around the meat and the pate.
5. Bake for about 20 to 30 minutes. Serve and enjoy.

Servings: 4
Calories: 307.5 |Net Carbs: 2.31 g| Fat: 22.66 g | Protein: 23.6 g

Cheeseburger Calzone

Ingredients
1 egg
1 c. of each:
   -Almond flour
   -Shredded mozzarella cheese
1 ½ lb. ground beef – lean
4 thick-cut bacon strips
½ yellow diced onion
4 dill pickle spears
8 oz. cream cheese – divided

1 c. shredded cheddar cheese
½ c. mayonnaise

Instructions
1. Set the oven temperature to 425°F. Use parchment paper to line a baking sheet. Slice the pickles into spears. Set aside for now.
2. Prepare the crust. Combine half of the cream cheese and the mozzarella cheese. Microwave for 35 seconds. Once it melts, add the almond flour and egg to make the dough. Set aside.
3. Cook the beef on the stove using medium heat. Cook the bacon (microwave for five minutes/stovetop). When cool, break into bits.
4. Dice the onion and add to the beef. Continue cooking until softened. Toss in the cheddar cheese, pickle bits, bacon, along with the rest of the cream cheese, and mayonnaise. Mix well.
5. Roll the dough onto the prepared baking tin. Add the mixture to the center. Fold the ends and side to make the calzone.
6. Bake until browned or about 15 minutes. Let it cool for ten minutes before slicing.

Servings: 8
Calories: 580 |Carbs: 3 g | Protein: 34 g | Fat: 47 g

Rib Eye Steak Salad

Ingredients
1 ribeye steak – 8 oz.
2 c. green salad mix
1 tbsp. of each:
    -Steakhouse seasoning
    -Olive oil
Pepper and salt to taste

1 t. wine vinegar

Instructions
1. Prepare the steak with the seasoning. Let it rest until cooled.
2. Arrange all of the salad fixings and add a sprinkle with the pepper and salt.
3. Toss and drizzle with the oil. Slice the steak into bite-sized strips.
4. Arrange the salad on two serving platters. Sprinkle the steak pieces on top.
5. Use your favorite dressing if desired, but count the carbs.

Servings: 2
Calories: 403 |Fat: 33 g | Net Carbs: 1.5 g | Protein: 25 g

Steak with Mushroom Port Sauce

Ingredients
10 oz. mushrooms
2 lb. Rib-eye steak
2 oz. heavy cream
1 tbsp. butter
4 oz. port wine
Salt & pepper

Instructions
1. Program the oven to 450°F.
2. Season the steak with pepper and salt. Add the butter to a cast iron skillet on high. Cook for two minutes on each side. Arrange the meat in a baking pan, and place it into the oven.
3. For medium rare, the internal temperature will be 135°F or a total of 12 minutes, flipping ½ through the cooking cycle. Cover with foil.

4. Pour the wine into the cooking pan to deglaze to bits. Add the cream and mushrooms. Cook until thickened.

Servings: 2
Calories: 984 | Protein: 102 g | Net Carbs: 6 g | Fat: 62 g

Seafood
Bacon Wrapped Scallops

Ingredients
12 of each:
   -Scallops
   -Thin bacon slices
   -Toothpicks
1 tbsp. oil
Pepper & salt to taste

Instructions
1. Use the high heat burner on the stovetop to warm up the oil.
2. Wrap each of the scallops with a strip of bacon and secure it tightly with a toothpick.
3. Add the scallops to the pan and fry for 2 ½ minutes for each side. Give it a shake or two of pepper and salt. Serve and enjoy as a snack or a luncheon.

Servings: 4
Calories: 204 | Protein: 27 g | Fat: 10 g| Net Carbs: 3 g

Cod in the Skillet

Ingredients
6 minced garlic cloves - divided
3 tbsp. ghee
4 cod fillets - 1/3 lb. each

Optional
  -Garlic powder
  -Salt

Instructions
1. Melt the ghee and add half of the garlic to a skillet.
2. Arrange the fillets in the pan using the medium-high heat setting. Sprinkle with the garlic, pepper, and salt.
3. When you turn it over, add the rest of the minced garlic. Continue cooking until it flakes easily.
4. Serve with some of the garlic ghee drippings from the pan.

Servings: 4
Calories: 160| Fat: 7 g | Carbs: 1 g |Protein: 21 g

Sesame Ginger Salmon
Ingredients
1 (10-oz.) salmon fillet
2 t. sesame oil
2 tbsp. of each
  -White wine
  -Soy sauce
1-2 t. minced ginger
1 tbsp. of each:
  -Rice vinegar
  -Sugar-free ketchup
  -Fish sauce – ex. Red Boat

Instructions
1. Combine all of the fixings in a Tupperware-type container (omit the ketchup, oil, and wine for now). Marinade them for about 1o to 15 minutes.
2. On the stovetop, prepare a skillet over high heat and pour in the oil. Add the fish when it's hot, skin side down.

3. Brown both sides for three to four minutes. Add the marinated juices to the pan and let it simmer when the fish is flipped.
4. Transfer the fish to a serving platter.
5. Add the wine and ketchup to the pan and simmer five minutes until it's reduced.
6. Serve the tasty salmon with your favorite veggie.

Yields: 2 Servings
Calories: 370 | Protein: 33 g | Net Carbs: 2.5 g | Fat: 23.5 g

Zesty Shrimp

Ingredients
½ lb. large shrimp
¼ c. olive oil
3 garlic cloves
Pepper and salt
1 lemon wedge

Instructions
1. Cook the garlic and cayenne along with the olive oil using medium heat on the stovetop. Peel and cook two to three minutes per side.
2. Flavor the shrimp with the pepper, salt, and lemon wedge.
3. Use the rest of the garlic oil as a dipping sauce.

Servings: 2
Calories: 335 | Net Carbs: 2.5 g | Protein: 22.5 g | Fat: 27 g

Chapter 7: Poultry and Pork Specialties

Bacon Chicken Ranch Casserole

Ingredients
8 slices bacon
2 lb. chicken breasts
1 lb. frozen spinach
¾ c. ranch dressing
3 minced garlic cloves
1 c. of shredded cheese each:
   -Mozzarella cheese – divided
   -Cheddar cheese - divided
Also Needed: 9x13 Casserole dish

Instructions
1. Cook the bacon and chop. Prepare the chicken and either shred or chop. Mince the garlic and thaw the spinach – squeezing to drain away the water.
2. Warm up the oven to 375°F.
3. Combine the bacon, chicken, garlic, spinach, ranch dressing, and ½ of thc shredded cheeses in a large mixing dish – stirring until well mixed.
4. Alternate layers or add together all of the fixings into the dish.
5. Top with the rest of the cheeses and bake for 15 minutes. Serve and enjoy!

Servings: 12
Calories: 332| Protein: 31 g | Net Carbs: 2 g | Fat: 22 g

Chicken Breast Salad with Honey Mustard Vinaigrette - Pressurized

Chicken Ingredients
1 c. cold tap water

1 (2/3 lb.) chicken breast

Ingredients for the Optional Quick Brining
2 tbsp. salt
2 c. cold tap water

Salad Ingredients
Grape tomatoes - halved
Field Greens

Honey Mustard Vinaigrette Salad Dressing Ingredients
3 tbsp. extra-virgin olive oil
1 tbsp. of each:
    -Balsamic vinegar
    -Honey
    -Dijon mustard
3 finely minced garlic cloves
1 pinch kosher salt
Also Needed: Pressure Cooker such as Instant Pot

Instructions
1. Remove all bones and skin from the breasts. Place the brine solution into a container along with the chicken, and place in the refrigerator to soak about 45 minutes. This will make the meat juicier.
2. Prepare the breasts by adding one cup of cold tap water into the pressure cooker. Arrange the chicken on the steamer rack and close for five minutes using the high-pressure setting. Natural release the pressure and open the lid. The internal temperature should be at least 163°F. Let it rest for five to ten minutes before slicing.
3. Prepare the dressing by combining all of the ingredients. Mix until emulsified.
4. Slice the chicken and add it on top of the greens and tomatoes. Give it a drizzle of the vinaigrette.
5. Serve and enjoy.

Servings: 2
Calories: 407 | Protein: 32 g | Net Carbs: 11 g | Fat: 25 g

Parmesan Chicken

Ingredients
1 ½ lbs. chicken breast – boneless
1 egg
¼ c. grated parmesan cheese
½ c. almond flour
½ t. kosher salt
½ t. garlic powder
1/8 t. cracked black pepper
½ t. dried basil
1 t. dried parsley
For Frying: 3 tbsp. olive oil

Casserole Ingredients
1 tbsp. olive oil
4 c. cooled spaghetti squash
½ tbsp. dried parsley
6 oz. fresh mozzarella
1/8 t. black pepper
1 ½ c. low-sugar salsa
For the Garnish: Chopped fresh basil
1 (9x13) baking pan

Instructions
1. Warm up the oven to 375°F.
2. Dice the chicken into two-inch bits. Beat the egg in a small container.
3. Mix the dry ingredients together in a medium bowl (dried parsley, almond flour, pepper, salt, parmesan cheese, and garlic powder).
4. Dip the chicken in the egg and then the breading mixture.

5. Warm up the oil in a skillet and cook the chicken until nicely browned. Drain on a towel-lined platter.
6. Combine the olive oil, spaghetti squash, salt, parsley, and pepper in a medium container. Toss well and add to the oven-safe baking dish.
7. Arrange the chicken over the squash, and empty the marinara sauce on the top.
8. Bake for about 30 minutes. Garnish with some chopped basil.

Servings: 8
Calories: 302 | Protein: 28 g | Net Carbs: 6 g | Fat: 8 g

Pesto Turkey Meatballs

Ingredients
¼ c. almond flour
1 lb. ground turkey
1 egg
¼ t. of each: Black pepper & salt
2 oz. fresh mozzarella
2 tbsp. pesto
For Frying: 2 tbsp. olive oil

Instructions
1. Use a medium container to combine the flour, turkey, salt, pepper, and egg. Stir until well incorporated. Shape into ten large meatballs.
2. Slice the mozzarella into ½-inch cubes. Flatten the balls in your hand and add the cube of cheese. Reshape the burger.
3. Use the low-medium heat setting on the stovetop, and add the oil to a saute pan. Fry for four minutes for each side until done.
4. Serve and enjoy.

Servings: 10 - 1 meatball (=) 1 Serving

Calories: 125 | Fat: 9 g | Net Carbs: 0.5 g |Protein: 10 g

Pork
Stuffed Pork Tenderloin on the Grill
Ingredients
2 lb. pork tenderloin or venison
½ c. of each:
    -Feta cheese
    -Gorgonzola cheese
1 t. chopped onion
2 tbsp. crushed almonds
2 minced cloves of garlic
½ t. of each:
    -Freshly cracked black pepper
    -Sea Salt

Instructions
    1. Warm up the grill. Create a pocket in the tenderloin.
    2. Combine the cheeses, almonds, onions, and garlic.
    3. Stuff the pork pocket and seal - using a skewer.
    4. Grill until done.

Servings: 1
Calories: 194 | Protein: 28.8 g | Net Carbs: 2.9 g | Fat: 6.2 g

Chapter 8: Tasty Side Dishes

Bacon & Cabbage Surprise

Ingredients
4 bacon slices
2 c. shredded cabbage
To Taste: Salt

Instructions
1. Place the cabbage in a pot with just enough water to cover. Boil for five to seven minutes.
2. Prepare the bacon and break into bits.
3. Add the bacon and salt to the cabbage and serve.

Yields: 1 Serving – 1 cup each
Calories: 346| Protein: 31 g | Net Carbs: 7 g | Fat: 9 g

Brussels Sprouts
Ingredients
2 tbsp. fresh lemon juice
¼ c. ghee – melted
½ t salt
1 lb. Brussels sprouts
Pinch freshly ground black pepper

Ingredient Variations
1 med. sliced white onion
2 crushed garlic cloves
¼ c. toasted pine nuts/cashews/flaked almonds
½ c. grated parmesan cheese

Instructions
1. Program the oven temperature to 400ºF.

2. Rinse and cut the sprouts into quarters. Add the melted ghee along with a drizzle of the lemon juice. Add any other ingredients you like.
3. Bake for 25-35 minutes. Stir occasionally.

Servings: 4
Calories: 179 |Protein: 4.2 g | Fat: 14.1 g |Net Carbs: 6.8 g

Cobb Salad

Ingredients
2 oz. chicken breast
2 bacon strips
1 hard-boiled egg
1 c. spinach
¼ avocado
½ Campari tomato
1 tbsp. olive oil
½ t. white vinegar

Instructions
1. Cook the chicken and bacon. Slice or shred the chicken.
2. Dice all of the fixings into bits and add them to a dish with the vinegar and oil. Toss gently and serve.

Servings: 1-2
Calories: 600| Protein: 43 g | Net Carbs: 3 g | Fat: 48 g

Collard Greens - Southern Style

Ingredients
1 ½ qt. water
1 ½ lbs. - ham hocks
4 lb. - collard greens
Optional: ½ t. crushed red pepper flakes
To Taste: Pepper & salt

¼ c. vegetable oil

Instructions
1. Pour the water into a large pot and add the ham hock using a tight-fitting lid. Lower the heat once it boils, and simmer for approximately 30 minutes.
2. Toss in the collard greens and the pepper flakes. Stir occasionally for about two hours. Pour in the oil and continue simmering for another 30 minutes.
3. Serve and enjoy with your favorite meat choice.

Servings: 6
Calories: 471 | Protein: 26.8 g | Net Carbs: 17.4 g | Fat: 34.3 g

Roasted Radishes

Ingredients
16 oz. red radishes
1 t. rosemary
4 tbsp. duck fat
To Taste: Pepper & salt

Instructions
1. Slice the radishes into halves. Add to a zipper bag with the seasoning and duck fat. Marinate about one hour.
2. Transfer to the baking pan and roast for 30 minutes.
3. Enjoy along with your favorite meat dish.

Servings: 5
Calories: 103.8| Net Carbs: 2 g | Fat: 10.2 g | Protein: 0.0 g

Spaghetti Squash with Cheese

Ingredients
1 tbsp. olive oil
2 c. cooked spaghetti squash

¼ c. whole milk ricotta cheese
Pepper and salt to taste
4 oz. mozzarella cheese
¼ c. basil pesto

Instructions
1. Program the oven setting to 375°F.
2. Cook and drain the squash, and add the oil with a sprinkle of salt and pepper. Spread it approximately two inches deep in a baking dish.
3. Scoop out the ricotta cheese and add on top of the squash. Cube the cheese and add it to the layers.
4. Bake until the cheese is melted or about ten minutes.
5. Place the squash on the counter to cool for about five minutes. Garnish with the pesto and serve.

Servings: 4
Calories: 207| Protein: 11 g | Net Carbs: 4.8 g | Fat: 17 g

Stuffed Peppers

Ingredients
2 sausage links
1 small onion
2 green peppers
2 oz. cream cheese
1 ½ oz. parmesan cheese
2 quail eggs/1 hen egg

Instructions
1. Program the oven temperature to 400°F.
2. Remove the skin from the sausage and crumble as it cooks in a skillet on the stovetop. Set aside.
3. Slice off the pepper tops and discard the seeds. Cut the heads off of the peppers along with the onions. Also, shred the parmesan into small bits.

4. Cook the onions and peppers in the skillet. Combine the peppers and onions with the sausage, cream cheese, and parmesan cheese.
5. Stuff the peppers and top it off with the egg or eggs.
6. Cook for 20 minutes and serve hot.

Servings: 2
Calories: 484 | Protein: 30 g | Net Carbs: 11 g | Fat: 35 g

Zucchini Fries
Ingredients
2 zucchinis
2 eggs
1 tbsp. salt
½ c. of each:
   -Ground almonds
   -Grated parmesan cheese
½ t. dried Italian herb seasoning – to taste

Instructions
1. Set the oven to 425°F.
2. Prepare a cooking tin with a parchment paper liner.
3. Slice the zucchini into three-inch lengths. Next, cut each of the pieces into nine fries. Arrange the pieces in a colander and give them a sprinkle of salt. Let them rest for about one hour until some of the liquid is removed.
4. In a small dish, whisk the eggs. Combine the Italian seasoning, almonds, and parmesan cheese in another bowl.
5. Rinse the salt from the zucchini and pat them dry with a few paper towels.
6. Dip the fries into the egg, then the almond coating. Put them on the prepared baking tin.
7. Bake about 25 minutes, turning halfway through. Enjoy!

Servings: 6
Calories: 98 | Protein: 8.9 g | Fat: 5.4 g |Net Carbs: 4.5 g

Chapter 9: Snacks & Desserts

Enjoy one of these tasty treats whenever your carbs allow!

<u>Blueberry Cream Pie</u>

Ingredients
1 cup raw of each:
    -Unsweetened shredded coconut
    -Unsalted sunflower seeds
¼ t. salt
¼ c. softened butter

Filling Ingredients
1 c. fresh/frozen blueberries
2 ½ t./1 envelope of gelatin
2 tbsp. of each:
    -Lemon juice
    -Water
¾ c. swerve sweetener
2 (8 oz.) pkg. softened cream cheese
½ t. liquid stevia
2 c. heavy cream – divided

Topping Ingredients
1 c. heavy cream
¼ c. blueberry mixture – reserved from the filling
½ t. vanilla liquid stevia
Also Needed: 8x8 baking dish

Instructions
1. Add all of the crust fixings in a food processor until combined. Coat the baking dish with a little non-stick cooking spray/oil. Add the crust.
2. Process the lemon juice and berries in the food processor until chopped.

3. Pour the water into a pan. Once it starts boiling, add the gelatin, stir, and set aside to cool.
4. In a stand mixer, add the cream cheese, ¾ cup of the berries, lemon stevia, and swerve – mixing until smooth. Stir in 1 cup of the heavy cream and blend two to three minutes. Drizzle with the gelatin and mix. Pour into the crust.
5. Add the other cup of heavy cream along with the rest of the berries and blend on the high setting in the mixture to form the topping.
6. Decorate the pie with the filling and chill in the fridge for two or three hours (overnight is best).
7. When ready to eat, decorate with a few berries.

Servings: 16
Calories: 305| Protein: 5.4 g | Fat: 29.9 g |Net Carbs: 3 g

Chocolate Chip Cookies

Ingredients
1 ¼ c. almond flour
2/3 c. sweetener/ swerve
1/8 t. sea salt – optional
1 ½ t. baking powder
1 tbsp. coconut flour
½ t. of each:
   -Vanilla extract
   -Molasses – optional
5 ½ tbsp. cold/room temperature butter
1 large egg
1/4 c. chopped pecans – optional
½ c. chocolate chips – sugar-free

Instructions
1. Use some parchment paper or silicone baking mats to line two baking sheets. Set the oven temperature to 325ºF.
2. Use a mixer to blend the sweetener and butter. Mix in the molasses, egg, and vanilla extract until well combined.
3. In another container, combine the two flours, sea salt, and baking powder -stirring until blended.
4. Fold in the pecans and chocolate chips. Arrange the cookie dough by the tablespoonful into the prepared pans. They should be 1 ½-inches apart.
5. Bake until the bottoms are browned or about 12-15 minutes.
6. Let them cool until firm and set (minimum 25 minutes).

Yields: 24 Cookies -1 of each per serving
Calories: 90 | Protein: 2 g | Net Carbs: 2 g | Fat: 8 g

Coconut Macaroons Fat Bombs

Ingredients
½ c. shredded coconut
¼ c. organic almond flour
2 tbsp. swerve
1 tbsp. of each:
    -Coconut oil
    -Vanilla extract
3 egg whites

Instructions
1. In a mixing bowl, blend the swerve, coconut, and almond flour until well combined.
2. Warm the oil in a saucepan and stir in the vanilla.
3. Place a medium-sized bowl in the freezer.
4. Combine the oil into the flour mixture, mixing well.

5. Put the whites of the eggs into the cold dish and whisk until
   stiff – foamy peaks are formed. Fold in the whites with the
   flour.
6. Scoop the mixture into the baking sheet/muffin cups.
7. Bake until the macaroons are lightly browned or about
   eight minutes.
8. Cool before placing on a serving dish.

Servings: 10
Calories: 46 | Fat: 5 g |Net Carbs: 0.5 g| Protein: 1.8 g

No-Bake Cheesecake

Ingredients for the Crust
2 tbsp. of each:
   -Melted coconut oil
   -Almond flour
   -Swerve Confectioner's/equivalent
   -Crushed salted almonds

Filling Ingredients
¼ c. swerve confectioner's/equivalent
1 t. gelatin
1 pkg. (8 oz.) cream cheese
½ c. unsweetened almond milk
1 t. vanilla extract

Instructions
   1. Prepare the crust by combining all of the fixings under the
      crust section. Place one heaping tablespoon into the bottom
      of dessert cups. Press the mixture down and set aside.
   2. Prepare the filling. Mix the sweetener and gelatin. Pour in
      the milk and stir (5 min.). Whip the vanilla beans and
      cream cheese with a mixer on medium until creamy. Add
      the gelatin mixture slowly until well incorporated.

3. Pour the mixture over the crust of each cup. Chill for three
    hours, minimum.

Servings: 6
Calories: 247 | Protein: 6.9 g | Net Carbs: 5 g | Fat: 25 g

Sesame Sugar Candied Pecans

Ingredients
2 c. pecans
5-8 tbsp. xylitol/Swerve
½ t. cinnamon
1 egg white
Optional: 1 t. blackstrap molasses
1 egg white
Flaky sea salt – to taste

Instructions
1. Line a rimmed baking tin with parchment paper. Warm up
    the oven to 250°F.
2. Combine the cinnamon, swerve, and molasses (if using) –
    mixing well.
3. Use an electric mixer to whip the eggs until soft peaks are
    formed.
4. Put the pecans into the sugar mixture and fold in the egg
    white.
5. Arrange the pecans (in a single layer) in the baking tin.
    Sprinkle with the salt.
6. Bake for 35-45 minutes. Check on them after about 10 to
    15 minutes and rotate them.
7. Cool completely. They get crispier when ready to eat.
8. Store up to one week in an air-tight container.

Servings: 10
Calories: 191 | Protein: 3 g | Net Carbs: 4 g | Fat: 19 g

In closing…

Thanks for reading your entire copy of The Keto Diet Guide for Beginners: Getting Started with the Low-Carb Ketogenic Diet. Let's hope it was informative and provided you with all of the tools you need to achieve your goals of following the keto diet and sticking to it.

The next step is to decide which tempting treat you should choose first. Just sit down and make a shopping list of all of the items you want to prepare for a couple of days. You don't have to stick to the daily plan as it is described. You have all of the nutritional counts for the diet in the chapters to follow throughout the book. You can mix and match as long as you stay within the limitations of 20 to 30 carbs daily or whatever your chosen method is for the keto plan.

Stay determined, and stand by your goals during your transition to ketosis. Follow the instructions and recipe methods. Before long, you will be able to quickly scan other recipes and know before you finish reading how healthy they are for you and your family.

The next step is to prepare your shopping list with all of the fixings needed for your menu plan. It will be a lot of fun to purge all of the 'toxins' you have been consuming over the years. All it takes is gathering your chosen meals and plan what's first!

Finally, if you found this book useful in any way, a review on Amazon is always appreciated!

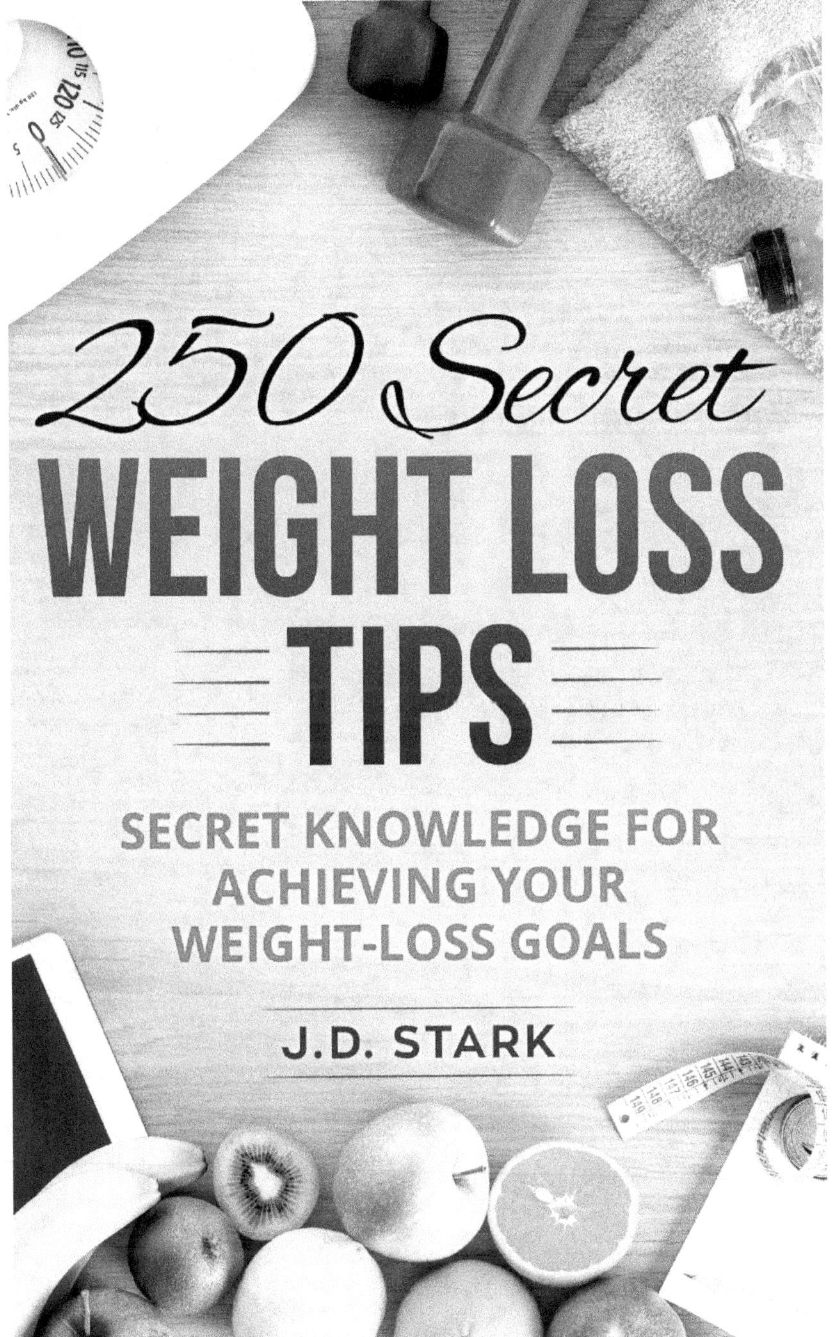

250 Secret
WEIGHT LOSS
TIPS
SECRET KNOWLEDGE FOR
ACHIEVING YOUR
WEIGHT-LOSS GOALS
J.D. STARK

250 Secret Weight Loss Tips

Secret Knowledge For Achieving Your Weight-Loss Goals

By J.D. Stark

http://www.jd-stark.com

Table of Contents

are mentioned are done without written consent and can in no way be considered an endorsement from the trademark holder.

Introduction

Congratulations on downloading this book and thank you for doing so. This book will give you important tips on losing weight and keeping your weight down.

We all want to have a fabulous looking body that makes people jealous. Yet, most people have to be content with using filters on their pictures posted on social networking sites. Most people would do anything to have the bodies they want. But very few have that body. Obesity or extra weight is a common problem. A simple search on the internet will show countless results telling numerous ways to reduce weight, but very few of them work effectively.

This book will not give you shortcut ways to lose weight. It brings to you 250 important tips to lose weight in a sustainable way. Here, 'sustainable' is the keyword because the biggest problem with most of the weight loss measures is sustainability. The amount of weight loss is generally lesser than the amount gained afterward. This book will explain some simple ways to lose weight in a slow and sustained manner.

It will walk you through the whole process in a methodical way.

Chapter 1 will tell you about the necessary mental preparations required for weight loss.

The 2nd chapter will give you an ideal meal plan that will help you in reducing your weight.

Chapter 3 will explain the impact of hunger and satiety hormones and the ways to bring them under control.

The 4th chapter will give you a list of food items that will help you in burning your fat faster.

Chapter 5 & 6 will discuss some workout tips and the ways to get the most out of them.

The 7th and 8th chapter will explain some important dietary rules and the necessary changes you will need to make in your lifestyle.

Chapter 9 & 10 will give you diet tips and also list the important food items to be included in your weight loss diet.

The last chapter will tell you some important rules that will help you in managing your weight effectively.

This book tries to deal with the issue through a different approach. It doesn't give you cheat sheet but encourages you to follow a dedicated path for long-term benefits.

You can gain a lot from this book and in turn lose weight too. It consists of simple 250 tips that will help you in tackling your weight issues easily and effectively.

There are plenty of books on this subject on the market, thanks again for choosing this one! Every effort was made to ensure it is full of as much useful information as possible, please enjoy!

Chapter 1: Mental Preparation for Weight Loss

1. Mentally Prepare Yourself

A fit body is everyone's desire. However, it takes a lot of hard work, determination and self-control to get one. You didn't exercise either of this and that has brought you to this stage in the first place. If you want to lose weight and look fit once again then you must prepare yourself mentally. It would indeed require a lot of sacrifices. You will have to be determined and plan things meticulously. Mental Preparation is the first step in losing weight.

2. Prepare a Chart of Your Current Diet

To lose weight you must start from the basic. To begin with, prepare a chart showing everything that you eat on regular basis. Do not leave out anything. No excuses here. There are plenty of resources available on the internet where you can get the estimate of calories you get from those items. Now, see the amount of calories you are consuming at present. This will help you in drawing an estimate of calories you would need to cut down. Be very meticulous in this step. Do not leave out anything at all.

3. Mark All the Places Where You Eat

Ideally, we all eat most of our food at home as breakfast and dinner are the big meals. But, home is not the only place where we eat. We also eat at our workplace, occasional parties, restaurants, etc. Calories consumed at these places also contribute equally to your weight. In fact, most of the times we eat fattening foods outside our homes. To cut down the calorie intake you will need to have a list of the places where you are most likely to eat. The number of calories you consume there. The number of times you are most likely to eat at those places in a week.

4. Check If You are an Impulsive Eater

Obese or overweight people tend to lose control on their eating habits. They tend to feel hungry when they see food. This is not entirely their fault. It is due to hormonal imbalance. Their mind is not able to differentiate between satiety and hunger. Inflammation in the fat cells is a major cause of this problem. This starts a vicious cycle of weight gain. The only way out is to eat consciously. Before every meal you must ensure that you are actually feeling hungry and not eating impulsively.

5. Analyze Your Emotions While Eating

Most overweight people loath eating but are unable to control the urge. This doesn't help them either. This depressing feeling pulls them down lower. It may even break their self-confidence and control. Before cutting down on calories, controlling such emotions is very important. You must write down the kind of emotions you feel while eating various kinds of foods. Guilt consciousness can be a real barrier. Grief is not going to pull you out of this fat. You must win over your mind before starting the battle with weight.

6. Write Down the Number of Calories You Burn in a Day

Although you may not realize it but every activity consumes energy. Hence, you are burning some part of the calories you consume in a day. For effectively losing weight you will have to burn more than you consume in a day. Write down all the physical activities you undertake in a day. From walking to your office to climbing the stairs of your apartment to walking your dog you must count all such activities.

7. Check Your Weight Regularly

There are many conflicting views about checking weight regularly. Some experts believe that regular checking your weight helps keep you aware of your weight loss goals. Others believe that regular checking doesn't help as you do not lose weight every day and hence this can demoralize you. Both are correct. However, even goods things must be done in moderation. You feel more encouraged when you achieve milestones. Regularly checking your weight is good. But, you won't lose weight on daily basis so daily checking can become an exercise in futility. Fix a day in the week to check your weight. A day when you are not working would be ideal for this.

8. Answer the Following Questions Honestly

a. How many meals do you have in a day?

b. How often do you eat out in a week?

c. what is your usual time between meals?

d. Are you a mindless eater?

e. Do you like junk food?

f. How many calories did you consume in the past week?

g. How many calories did you burn in the past week?

h. Do you like watching TV while eating?

i. What is the amount of time between your dinner and going to bed?

j. Which is the easiest meal to skip for you?

You must think about these questions very seriously and give honest answers. Be definite about the replies. There are no right or wrong answers to these questions. The answer to these questions would change as you move ahead in your weight loss efforts. Ponder over them and write your answers down.

9. Follow a Sustainable Weight Loss Plan

Setting big goals and aiming to shed several pounds of fat is a week or month is an unsustainable plan. Such goals are never met. You will only get disappointment in the end. Set achievable goals of few pounds a month. Remember that you not only have to lose that weight but maintain it too. While you are at it, you will also have to carry on your life as normal. Things like going to work and enjoying life cannot be put on the backburner.

10. Start Making Small Changes at First

Start by making small changes in your lifestyle. Cut down on eating out. Start putting more fruits and salads in your diet. Slowly and gradually start eliminating processed and sugary foods from your diet. You should do this slowly. Do not do everything at once as you'll start feeling pathetic. Such enthusiasm doesn't last long and you'll quickly return to your normal routine. Therefore, it is important to bring such changes slowly. First, bring more fruits and vegetables into your diet. Then start cutting out the sugary foods. Always remain conscious of the number of calories you consume in a day. Increase the number of fasting hours in a day.

Chapter 2: The Meal Plan

When it comes to weight loss 'one plan fits all' doesn't work. Every person has individual needs. Your meal plan must fulfill your energy requirements while helping in weight loss. However, the higher the number of meals you consume the greater are the chances of high-calorie intake. You must devise a plan to cut down the number of meals.

The Ideal Day Plan

11. Begin Your Day with Exercise

Burning more calories should be your goal. When you wake up your body has been in the fasting state for 7-8 hours. Exercise in this state is the best for burning calories quickly. You may feel hungry in the beginning but slowly you'll get used to it. Do some form of exercise daily. Go for a walk, do yoga, run on treadmill or jog. These activities will not only help you lose weight but will also make you feel refreshed. You will feel energetic and positive for the whole day. Feeling positive is very important for losing weight.

12. Drink Lemon, Honey and Water

Begin your day by drinking honey, lemon and water. Lemon and honey help in melting down your fat. It will also help in detoxifying your body. It is a low calorie drink that will aid your digestion and also act as natural diuretic. This simple drink has lots of benefits and it is very easy to prepare. By the time you get to the breakfast table this drink will keep you fresh.

13. Have a Healthy Breakfast

Some experts strongly recommend a heavy breakfast. It is touted as the most important meal of the day. However, breakfast is only the first meal of the day. You have been in the fasting state for a prolonged duration and therefore this meal should be healthy. You must not have a very heavy breakfast or you'll keep feeling lethargic the whole day. In fact you must have a healthy breakfast that consists of fruits, cereals, and whole grains. Eating protein-rich foods is especially good for breakfast as they make you feel fuller quickly. Try to have egg-whites, cereals, whole grains, skimmed milk, sprouts and fruits in your breakfast.

14. Sugar Free Beverages Only Before Lunch

You must ensure that you do not consume beverages with added sugar. Soda, or coffee with sugar will give you unwanted amount of calories. You must avoid them at all costs. While at work you can consume black coffee to avoid any sort of hunger pangs. It will not only keep you satiated but alert too.

15. Have a Moderate Lunch

Lunch is the trickiest meal of the day. Keeping a strict control on the number of calories you consume at lunch is very important. People tend to eat with colleagues at lunch and to eat out. This way a lot of unwanted calories get added. You should make it a practice to take your lunch from home. It can have fruits and vegetables. Homemade preparations will have a lot less fat and calories than the food available at fast food chains and cafeterias. Try to include probiotic drinks, salads and protein-rich foods in this meal.

16. Have Fruits or Sprouts as an Evening Snack

Evening snacks are the unwanted calories that are completely avoidable. However, some people can't resist food for very long. If you also fall in this category, then eating fruits or sprouts will be the best option. They help ease your hunger and make you feel satiated without adding too many calories. Too much indulgence at this point can be counterproductive.

17. Dinner- The Lighter the Better

Your dinner should be the lightest meal of your day. Ideally, you must take your dinner at least 4 hours before going to bed. This will help in proper digestion of this meal. However, for all practical reasons we know that it isn't possible these days. To compensate that, you must take your dinner as early as possible as keep it as light as manageable. Eat a lot of fiber-rich food for dinner, including lots of salads. Foods that are rich in protein but low on fat, sugar and carbohydrates must be included in the dinner.

18. Go for a Post-dinner Walk

A light walk after dinner is one of the healthiest practices. This walk is beneficial in many ways. You will be able to digest your food better with the help of this walk. A light walk helps you in going over the activities of the day and also gives you time to plan for the next day. It gives you quality time for self-introspection or having a healthy chat with your partner. It makes you feel better.

Feeling better and relaxed is an important part of losing weight.

19. Limit Sugar and Sweet Intake

Sugar and sweets are unhealthy. You must avoid them as much as possible. Eating sugar may give you an instant burst of energy but it leads to insulin resistance in the long run. You will gain weight faster and it'll get difficult to control calorie intake. The best way to avoid sugar is to have fruits instead. The fruits also contain fructose but that is easy to break down. It doesn't lead to insulin resistance in the body.

20. Avoid Drinking Water with Meals

This is a very simple yet important advice. The biggest reason for most problems in our body is poor digestion. Drinking water while eating dilutes the digestive juices. The process of digestion gets slow and problems like acidity, bloating, and indigestion emerge. This may also interfere with the proper functioning of the liver. It is a very important organ for metabolization of fat in the body. Therefore the chances of poor fat metabolization increase.

Chapter 3: Bell the Cat- Bring Ghrelin Under Control

The biggest hurdle in front of weight loss measures is controlling hunger. Overweight people seem to have frequent hunger pangs. Their body doesn't seem to get enough energy. It needs food at regular intervals. The real problem lies with the improper management of the 'Hunger Hormone'. Ghrelin is an appetite-increasing hormone. Our gut releases it when it gets empty. Its levels are highest when your stomach is completely empty and the lowest after meals. Ghrelin levels also increase when you are in stressful or sad state. This is a major way depression contributes to weight gain.

21. Understand the Relationship Between Ghrelin and Leptin

Ghrelin is the 'Hunger hormone' and Leptin is the 'Satiety hormone'. Your body needs to have a delicate balance of both. Inflammation of fat cells is common in overweight people that leads to leptin insensitivity. This means that your body keeps sending the message that it's full but your brain doesn't recognize it. Your body keeps releasing Ghrelin and you lose control on your appetite. Managing both these hormones is important.

22. Adopt Smart Dietary Choices to Bring Harmony

The right mix of healthy life choices like balanced diet, exercise, proper sleep and stress management can help you. This will increase Ghrelin and Leptin sensitivity and you're weight management will become easier.

23. Don't Overdo Calorie Restriction

When people begin weight loss they get overenthusiastic and exercise extreme calorie restriction. This can be counterproductive. Eating nutrient-dense and fiber-rich foods should be your goal. You must not have processed food in your diet.

24. Eat the Right Amount of Protein

A protein-rich diet can help in controlling hunger pangs. A study published in American Journal of Clinical Nutrition states that high-protein diets help in suppressing Ghrelin release for longer periods. You will feel fuller much faster and keep feeling satiated for longer.

25. Exercise

High-Intensity Interval Training is the best when it comes to Ghrelin control. Several studies have demonstrated that burst training decreases the ghrelin release. This means that you'll feel less inclined to eat after high-intensity workouts like sprinting and cycling. It has dual benefits. It helps in controlling hunger and also aids weight loss.

26. Get a Good Night's Sleep

Sleep is very helpful in managing the ghrelin release properly. Sleep deprivation can lead to increased levels of ghrelin in the body. The longer the period of undisturbed sleep the better will be the hunger management.

27. Manage Your Stress

Ghrelin release is directly related to your stress levels. When you are sad, depressed or stressed you tend to feel more inclined towards eating. This even gives a boost to mindless eating habit. You must adopt methods like meditation to manage your stress levels. Spending time outdoors and walking are some of the activities that also help in managing stress. You should also include anti-inflammatory foods in your diet to decrease stress.

28. Avoid Processed Foods

Processed foods contribute a lot towards the increase in ghrelin levels. Processed food is calorie dense and our system is hardwired to enjoy such foods. It relishes such foods and doesn't send the signals to stop and ultimately you consume high quantities of such foods. This doesn't help in any way. You must avoid such foods and consume nutrient-dense foods.

29. Bring Anti-inflammatory Foods into Your Diet

The best way to bring the ghrelin and leptin hormones under control is to cure chronic inflammations. They are the root cause of most of the problems. Anti-inflammatory foods can help you in curing such inflammations. They help in increasing sensitivity towards such hormones and you start feeling fuller at a faster rate.

30. Remain Hydrated

Water is the basic need of life. It is important for most of our body functions. Besides other things, it can also help in fighting hunger pangs and reducing weight. You must drink the right amount of water and keep yourself hydrated at all times.

Chapter 4: Include Fat Burning Foods in Your Diet

It takes a lot of effort to lose weight. You will have to take several measures and exercise great self-control. The process is never very fast and painless. However, there are some specific food items that can help you burn fat faster.

31. Bone Broth

When it comes to fat burning foods nothing beats bone broth. It is full of amino acids that prevent muscle breakdown while accelerating fat burn. It increases your metabolism and also detoxifies your body.

32. Chicken

A vegetarian diet is great for losing weight but it can get really difficult to switch instantly to such a diet. Chicken is the best option in such cases. It not only pleases your taste buds but also provides a sufficient amount of protein. It'll keep you satiated and energized.

33. Apple Cider Vinegar

This is a magic formula when it comes to reducing appetite. A small amount of apple cider vinegar before a meal can help you in feeling fuller much faster. This way you'll consume less food. It also detoxifies your body and balances the pH in your stomach.

34. Cayenne Pepper

It is one of the best spices to bring flavor to your plate. This mild pepper will spice up your food and also increase your body's ability to burn fat. It boosts your metabolism and helps your weight loss efforts. You can use it in your diet in a number of ways.

35. Chia Seeds

Chia seeds are the best if you want to reduce your hunger pangs and sugar cravings and increase immunity. These seeds are an excellent source of Omega-

3 fatty acids and very rich in antioxidants. They provide large amount of good cholesterol and also help burn fat faster.

36. Cruciferous Vegetables

Cruciferous vegetables like cauliflower, kale and Brussels sprouts are nutrient dense. They are packed with calories and give your body the required nutrition while burning fat. You must include these vegetables in your diet for faster weight loss.

37. Grapefruit

It works wonders in burning fat and also helps in breaking down sugar faster. You must include grapefruit in your breakfast or drink grapefruit juice as a refreshing beverage. It increases your metabolism and curbs your craving for food.

38. Coconut Oil

One of the biggest reasons for abnormal weight gain is uncontrolled thyroid, especially in women. Coconut oil is one of the best and healthiest fats for such a situation. It helps in decreasing body weight as well as body fat. It helps in regulating the thyroid hormone. You can accelerate fat burning by including coconut oil when cooking food.

39. Green Leafy Vegetables

There is no hidden secret about the benefits of eating green leafy vegetables. They are simply great for your health. They are packed with vitamins and minerals. Apart from that, they are nutrient dense and help in burning calories.

40. Whey Protein

Whey protein is great for decreasing body fat and increasing muscle buildup. It keeps you feeling fuller for longer and reduces your calorie intake. It helps you in keeping your blood sugar levels stable while providing high energy level for long periods of time.

Chapter 5: Workout Tips

Exercise is one of the best and fastest ways to reduce weight. It keeps you fit and makes you feel better.

Some of the top ways are:

41. Yoga

Yoga is one of the easiest ways to lose weight effectively. It is safe and easy to perform. You can practice it in groups as well as alone. It not only helps you in losing weight and cutting down belly fat but also provides several other health benefits. Yoga can help you lose weight and also keep it under control with great ease.

42. Crunches

Crunches are effective and efficient. They help you lose belly fat and weight. The higher the number of crunches you perform the better your shape will be. The best thing about crunches is that you do not need to go anywhere to perform them. You can easily do crunches at your home. There can be no excuse to skip the daily routine of crunches if you are really inclined to lose weight.

43. Planks

Planks are easy to perform and require very little guidance. You can easily do several sets of planks along with crunches and other exercises daily. They help in reducing weight and belly fat. You'll have toned muscles and a great body. You must perform several sets of planks every day for faster weight loss.

44. Lunges

Lunges especially forward lunges are great for toning muscles and weight loss. They keep you in shape and make the weight loss journey worthy in all respects. Your core muscles will get the required exercise and remain fit. They are really great for your thighs and legs. They must be a part of your weight loss regimen as no one would want to look like an empty sack after losing weight. These exercises keep your body toned and healthy.

45. High-intensity Exercises

High-intensity exercises are the best for losing overall weight faster. You can burn a lot of calories in each session and build muscles. These are the best for people who want to shed dozens of pounds faster. However, it is important to understand that if you want to take a long-term view then going slow on high-intensity workouts will be the best. People tend to lose momentum over a period of time as these exercises are physically very demanding. Going to a nearby gym would be the best option for these exercises.

46. Cardio Exercises

Cardio exercises are the best for maintaining a healthy body. You can use cardio exercises like cycling, swimming, running, rowing for both low and high-intensity exercises. Choose the tempo that suits you the best and maintain it in the long run. These exercises have a long-term positive impact on your overall health and weight. You can easily lose weight through these exercises and maintain it without much effort.

47. Walking and Jogging

These are two age old tried and tested ways to remain fit and lose weight. They are suitable for people from all age groups. They keep you fresh and healthy. You will lose weight and also remain fit for longer. If you have a sedentary lifestyle where you are required to sit in front of a desk for longer periods then walking around often in your office can also help a lot. It will keep you fresh and also give exercise to your muscles. Remember, even short walks help in burning calories and therefore every walk contributes towards your weight loss efforts.

48. Bear Crawls

Bear crawls are great for strengthening your arms, shoulders and chest. They works on your core muscles and also burn calories. You can easily lose weight and keep your muscles toned by including them in your daily exercise routine.

49. Jumping

Jumping is a high impact exercise. This workout helps you burn body fat faster. It gives you a great energy boost and you will feel light after short jumping sessions. You can perform several jumping exercises like rope jumping, box squat jumps, step up jumps in your workout.

50. Running

Running is one of the best exercises to burn calories and keep your heart healthy. It helps you in losing a lot of calories and burning the adamant belly fat. You can choose your own pace and time for running and keep increasing it over time.

All these exercises are great for sustainable weight loss. There are several other high-intensity workouts that can help you in losing weight faster. However, the problem with most of them is that you lose the impetus and motivation after a short period of time. You lose weight faster with them but as soon as you get a bit relaxed you start gaining weight even faster. These exercises can be done at a steady rate for a much longer period. They do not need any special preparation or time. You can take them up at your own pace and continue them for sustainable periods.

Chapter 6: Some Important Workout Secrets

51. Schedule Your Workouts Carefully

One of the most important steps to effectively lose weight is to include it in your daily schedule. If you are serious about weight loss then it will need your time. When you plan your days and weeks keep the time slot for daily exercise without fail. They are as important as your business meetings. You can't ignore them even for a day if you are serious about weight loss.

52. Take Out Time for Short Exercise Breaks Throughout the Day

Doing an hour of exercise in the morning can take a toll on you. You do not need to do all the exercise in one stretch. Plan your day in a way that you get exercise in short intervals and they'll have the same impact on your weight. For instance, do crunches, lunges and planks along with some high-intensity workout in the morning. Then plan some short walks in the day during your lunch hour. Light exercises in the evening and a brisk walk after dinner can give you great benefits. You'll lose weight much faster and will be able to maintain it without great efforts.

53. Don't Miss Exercise Even While You are Travelling

Short breaks like travelling to other cities for work or pleasure can become a great impediment in weight loss efforts. Such things shouldn't become a hurdle in your way. You can plan these exercises even while you are travelling as you do not need equipment or accessories. Never miss on these exercise while you are out of town.

54. Bring Variations in Your Routine

Change can spice things up in life and it is equally true for exercises. You do not need to stick to any single workout for weight loss. You can add variations as per your convenience to keep things interesting. Experiment with pace and time in running. Increase time of exercises and add more routines. You can also plan some exercises for alternate days and others for the remaining days of the week. The important thing is to keep doing them without breaks.

55. Take Interest

The biggest reason for leaving exercises is that people start losing interest in them. This proves to be a great setback. It must be avoided by all means. You must ensure that you keep exercising without substantial breaks. If there are particular routines that are difficult for you then choose other routines that suit you more. Doing something is always better than doing nothing. Adjust the difficulty level of exercises as per your ability.

56. Remain Conscious of Budgetary Constraints

Some people join expensive gyms and clubs for faster weight loss but then leave it soon as they find it too expensive. This is a wrong approach towards weight loss. Your weight loss efforts don't need to be a drain on your pocketbook. If your budget doesn't allow joining high cost gyms and clubs then start exercising at home. Do yoga or light exercises as they are equally beneficial in the long run. Do not chase after faster gains. Look for sustainable methods of weight loss. You can easily lose weight through yoga, cardio and aerobic exercises too. Methods like walking, running, hiking cost no money at all and give equally great results.

57. Music Keeps You Tuned

Listening to music while exercising is a great way to maintain them. It keeps you focused and you work out for longer. While exercising choose the kind of music you like and focus on your workout. This way you'll be able to work out for longer without getting bored.

58. Join a Group

A little motivation from others and a push is necessary. You can get both when you work out in a group. You can join yoga clubs or form a group of friends to work out together. This will help you in getting up daily and doing exercise. Your routine wouldn't break and you'll be able to exercise even on those days when you want to skip it. Watching others lose weight faster also gives a motivation to work harder. It provides you the supporting environment and brings you in the mood.

59. Start Your Day with a Workout

There are several benefits of working out first thing in the morning. First, the body and mind are fresh in the morning and hence you can work out great. Second, at this time your body is producing the highest amount of hGH that leads to faster weight loss. Third, starting the day with a workout builds the momentum and keeps you fresh and light for the whole day. It gives a great start to your day and you'll feel lighter and happier. Even if you miss the short workouts later in the day there would be no guilt pangs as you would have done most of it in the morning .

60. Add Weightlifting in Your Routine

Weightlifting is a great way to give a big push to your weight loss efforts. Experts believe that weightlifting not only accelerates weight loss but also helps in shedding belly fat. It is a faster way to lose fat from all over your body. Your muscles will strengthen and you'll feel lighter.

Chapter 7: Important Dietary Rules

61. Eat Food Slowly

Eating your food slowly is very important. When you eat food really quick your brain isn't able to assess the amount of food ingested. You eat more than required. Eating slow will make you feel fuller even with low amount of food. Your calorie intake will reduce.

62. Wait for Some Time Before Taking the Second Serving

If you need a second helping and aren't feeling satiated yet then wait for some time. There is a greater likeliness that you wouldn't feel hungry after few minutes. By this time your body realizes that it doesn't need more food and the appetite vanishes.

63. Fix a Place for Eating

This may sound weird but it is important. We generally eat at the dining table but that's not the rule. We also eat sitting in front of the TV, in the kitchen or even in the bedroom at times. If we develop a habit of only eating at the dining table, then the habit of mindless eating can be controlled.

64. Never Watch TV while Eating

Watching TV while eating may lead to consumption of more food as you are paying less attention to the food than TV. Do not do anything else like talking, reading, watching TV or surfing your mobile phone. Focus on your food and its quantity.

65. Use Smaller Plates

Smaller plates for eating lead to less food per serving. This is a great way to limit the quantity of food you eat.

66. Don't Bring Extra Food to the table

Keeping too much food on the table also leads to consumption of greater amount of food. Only bring foods in your plates and bring more later if you need. Most likely you'll not need extra food.

67. Don't Go Outside with an Empty Stomach

Going out of your home with an empty stomach opens the chances of eating out. You will have no control on the amount of calories eaten. Always eat before you leave home so that you do not feel like eating unhealthy food outside.

68. Avoid Fast Food Completely

Fast food available in the market is very unhealthy. It is laden with processed sugar and fats. You can throw your aim of losing weight out of the window if you cannot put a stop to eating fast food.

69. Include Foods in Your Diet That Require Chewing

Foods that need to be chewed for long give you a feeling of satisfaction faster. You feel fuller even after eating small quantities. It is important to include such food items in your diet.

70. Include More and More Salads in Your Diet

Salads are full of fiber and good for health. Beside, eating salads will reduce your appetite and you'll consume less calories and fat.

71. Don't Begin Your Day with Tea or Coffee

Caffeine-rich products are unhealthy, give a bad start to your day, and it induce stress. Start your day with a glass of plain water or water with lemon and honey. It will keep you refreshed and detoxify your body.

72. Adopt Intermittent Fasting

Develop a shorter eating window for yourself. The longer you fast, the faster will be your weight loss. Begin eating late in the morning and take two or three meals of the day at shorter intervals. This will give you a longer fasting window. Your body will be able to process food better and you'll lose weight.

73. Avoid Eating Anything Late in the Evening

The earlier you eat in the evening, the better. The food consumed closer to bedtime doesn't get enough time for processing. You should eat several hours before you go to sleep.

74. Avoid a Carbohydrate-Rich Diet

Food items with high carbohydrate content and less fiber are bad for your health. They increase your appetite and blood glucose levels. Eat nutrient-dense food items for faster weight loss.

75. Eat More and More Fruits and Vegetables

Fruits and vegetables are the best for weight loss. They are rich in fiber and antioxidants. These are important ingredients for effective weight loss.

76. Decrease the Intake of White Items

Food items like potato, sugar, white rice are unhealthy and their intake should be limited. These items are calorie dense and lead to faster weight gain.

78. Include Whole Grains in Your Diet

Whole grains are the best when it comes to a healthy diet. They are rich in fiber and vitamins. You must consume whole grains for faster weight loss. They improve your gut health and lead to better processing of food.

79. Use Skimmed Milk and Probiotics

Skimmed milk is the best when it comes to dairy. It gives you the required protein without the malicious fat. Probiotics are easy to digest and improve your gut health.

80. Choose to Drink Water when Thirsty

Avoid drinking carbonated beverages like soda as they have added sugar and calories. Even the zero calorie drinks are not free from bad things. They'll lead to faster weight gain than anything else. Whenever you feel thirsty only drink water.

Chapter 8: Some Lifestyle Changes for Weight Loss

81. Identify Your Triggers

Some mental conditions contribute a lot towards weight gain. Some people eat more when stressed others when sad. You must remain conscious of such situations and avoid eating in them.

82. Avoid Mindless Eating

Mindless eating is dangerous. You can consume more calories than required through this habit. Avoid munching food without proper hunger. You can start chewing gum in such situations when you feel like eating anything.

83. Skip Dressing Your Salads

People like dressing up their salads with oil, cheese and sauces. These items add fat and calories to your food and take away the health benefits. Keep your salads as simple as possible.

84. Use Cooking Sprays in Place of Cooking Oil

Cooking sprays add less fat to your food and avoid burning food. They are a healthy alternative to cooking oil. You can reduce your fat intake this way.

85. Shop the Perimeter of the Grocery Stores

Most of the grocery stores have healthy food items in the perimeter and processed food items in the center rows. So try to restrict your grocery shopping to the outer circle of the stores.

86. Walk Whenever Possible

Walking is a good exercise. You must try to walk as much as possible. Park your vehicle as far as possible from your destination so that you get a chance to walk. This will help in burning more calories.

87. Use Stairs as Much as Possible

Using lifts and elevators has become a habit these days. But, the good old habit of climbing the stairs not only gives you good exercise of lungs but also burns a lot of calories. Try using the stairs whenever possible.

88. Develop Hobbies That Require Physical Labor

Activities like gardening or cleaning your house are labor intensive. They give you a lot of exercises and keep you engaged. Developing such hobbies can also help you in your weight loss efforts.

89. Take Part in Athletic Events

Corporate lifestyle takes away the chances for physical activity. It makes us lethargic. Try to take part in athletic events organized by your company or club. It helps you in becoming active and losing weight.

90. Cut Down Your TV Time

Watching TV can make you inactive. You start feeling tired faster and feel hungry frequently. The commercials of food items provoke you to eat. Cut down your TV time and use it for physical activities.

91. Walk Your Dog More Often

Walking your dog is also a good physical activity. It gives you an opportunity to venture out of your home and burn some extra calories. Start walking your dog more often. This will also help in bonding better with your pet.

92. Bring Your Treadmill to Your Living Room

Most of us buy treadmills but tend to stop using them as they are kept in some secluded corners. Bring them to your living room or a place you spend most of your time. This will give you greater motivation to use them.

93. Set Small Milestones

It is very important to remain motivated. Set smaller milestones of weight loss. Every little achievement will help you to work harder.

94. Weigh Yourself at Regular Intervals

Weighing yourself everyday may not be very motivating and effective but weighing yourself weekly can be. You will be able to see the success of your efforts this way. Use your weighing scale every week to see if your efforts are bringing desired results. If they aren't then start working a bit harder.

95. Be Consistent

One of the biggest problem with weight loss is that people are not consistent in their efforts. They start with great zeal but then the downward slope starts. Be consistent in your weight loss efforts for satisfactory results.

96. Keep Your Fridge Clean

Do not pack your fridge with unnecessary food items. This gives an opportunity to munch on unnecessary food items when you feel like it. The lower the amount of items in your fridge the greater are the chances of avoiding unhealthy or excessive intake of food.

97. Avoid Eating at Night

Not working till late at night is not a luxury for most of us. Excessive work pressure makes us work till late. This is the time when hunger pangs trouble the most. Avoid eating at such times. When feeling very hungry limit yourself to coffee without sugar. It will curb your hunger without adding calories.

98. Eat Only When Really Hungry

Impulsive eating is bad. Do not start eating whenever you feel. Let your body actually demand food. It'll be difficult in the beginning but you can train your body and mind to do that with some practice. This will limit your calorie intake.

99. Blue Color Plates

Blue is hunger suppressant. Blue color plates can help you in curbing your appetite. Flashy bright color plates do the opposite.

100. Eat in Front of Mirror

Studies have shown that eating in front of mirrors curbs appetite. When you see eating yourself for too long you stop feeling hungry. This can help you if you have a habit of eating more.

101. Walk for at Least 45 Minutes in a Day

This is a fairly easy target to achieve. The total walking time in a day is usually around this much. Try to record the amount of time you walk in a day. You can do this with the help of several devices available in the market or even with applications on your smartphone. If you are walking any less than increase the time. This will increase the number of calories you burn.

102. Never Buy Prepared Meals

Prepared meals available in the market are full of calories, salt, unhealthy fats and processed sugar. These are unhealthy and add a lot of calories to your meal. Try to cook all your meals at home. You'll eat healthy and fresh food with known calories.

103. Read the Labels of Food Items Carefully

This one habit can help you in reducing a large amount of calories and fats from your food. Do not buy food products mindlessly. Carefully scan the number of calories and fats in the food items you buy.

104. Drink Water Before Eating

Drinking water before meals makes you feel fuller much faster. You will not over eat and feel much more satisfied even with small quantities of food.

105. Get Rid of Your Older Clothes

When you start losing weight getting rid of your older clothes gives great motivation. It keeps you inspired to maintain the weight and lose much more. So keep cleaning your wardrobe frequently.

106. Stay Away from Kitchen for at Least 12 Hours

Try to stay away from your kitchen as long as possible. This way you'll be able to control the amount of food you eat. Restricting your food intake will become easier if your reduce the number of trips to the kitchen.

107. Go for a Walk before Dinner

We all know that a brisk walk after dinner is good for health. However, a walk before dinner is even better for weight loss. A walk before dinner raises your body temperature and hence your appetite reduces. Your food intake reduces in turn and you consume less calories.

108. Plan Active Outings on Weekends

We all need a break and weekends are an ideal time for that. However, planning barbeque parties can be an unhealthy break for your health. Instead, plan active outings on weekends. You'll be able to gel better with your near and dear ones and also burn a lot more calories in the process. Go for hiking, games and other physically taxing fun activities.

109. Count Your Steps

Using pedometers can be the best solution to keep track of the amount of distance you cover on foot in a day. It will keep you motivated to walk more. You'll remain active this way and burn more calories.

110. Try to Eat at Home

Eating out sometimes becomes unavoidable. However, it shouldn't become a habit. You can't control the number of calories and fats present in the food. It generally contains high amount of both for adding taste. You must try to eat as much as possible at home.

111. Switch to Simple Coffee

Coffee is a refreshing beverage and there can be no argument over it. However, going for the richer variants that contain more milk and sugar may not be the best for your health. Stick to simple black coffee as it is low calorie, refreshing and healthy drink.

112. Eat Most Calories before Lunch

Our body needs time to process the calories we consume in a day. The later we do that the longer it takes to get processed. If we consume the calories while we are still active then they get processed as energy or else they'll get converted into fat. Therefore, it is important to consume most of the calories prior to your lunch so that there is time to process them. The more you eat in dinner the higher the chances of weight gain.

113. Brush Your Teeth After Meals

Brushing your teeth is important part of oral hygiene. But, it is also has an impact on your eating habits. After brushing your tendency to eat anything reduces. You can easily avoid mindless eating. You must make a habit of brushing after meals and especially after dinner.

114. Start Experimenting with Cooking

Cooking is a very engaging activity. It keeps you interested in your food and you can also have complete control over it. This way chances of consuming unhealthy items and extra calories decrease. Once you start enjoying the process, you'll get complete control on the kind of food you eat.

115. Pack Your Lunch Daily

Eating out for lunch is a common practice. It is efficient and easy. However, it isn't healthy in the same manner. You must develop the habit of taking your lunch from your home. It can be anything from an assortment of fruits and vegetable salads to sprouts to healthy preparations.

116. Enjoy Using the Exercise Ball

There is a great amount of time when we are idling in front of the TV or computer screens. Spending this time on an exercise ball can not only make the time more engaging but can also help you in burning up some extra calories.

117. Take Interest in Adventure Sports

Everyone has a wild side. We like things that thrill us and give an adrenaline rush. Adventure sports have this quality. They not only make us feel more alive but also help us in burning a lot of extra calories. Plan adventure sports regularly.

118. Stop Smoking

Smoking causes cancer and it is known to everyone. But, it can also force you to crave for high fat foods. This leads to unnecessary weight gain. Smoking decreases the serotonin levels in your brain and you have to look for high-fat foods for taste. You can enjoy even low calorie foods if you stop smoking.

119. Go Easy on Alcohol

There are many reasons not to drink alcohol and weight gain is among one of the most important ones. Besides giving you a pot belly it also adds a lot of calories to your diet. Alcohol contain 7 calories per gram and therefore the higher the alcohol the greater is calorie intake. It also damages your liver which is the main organ for metabolizing fat and processing energy.

120. Beware of High Blood Pressure

Weight gain is among the chief causes of high blood pressure but high blood pressure can also lead to unnatural weight gain. Most of the blood pressure drugs contain salts that lead to weight gain. Keeping your blood pressure in check can keep you away from them.

121. Go for Local Harvest instead of Canned Food

Canned food will always fare low when compared to local harvest. Local harvest is natural and free from added preservatives, salts and flavors. It gives you the right amount of nutrition and also helps your community. Give preference to it for faster weight loss.

122. Stop Drinking Soda

All kinds of soda or carbonated beverages may seem refreshing and tempting but they neither quench your thirst nor provide health benefits. They simply add calories to your body. Excess amount of refined sugar causes the extra harm. You must avoid them as much as possible.

123. Eat Organic Foods

Organic foods that are free from pesticides and herbicides are great for health. The side effect of these chemicals can be plenty and they also cause severe hormonal changes that may lead to weight gain. Switching to organic foods can help in avoiding the intake of these harmful chemicals.

124. Avoid Trans-fat Foods

Trans-fat is simply bad. It must be avoided in all circumstances. Period.

125. Lower Your Saturated Fat Intake

Higher intake of saturated fats can be detrimental to your weight loss efforts. It increases your total cholesterol levels and also adds a lot of calories to your diet. You should cut down your daily saturated fat intake and limit it to less than 7% of your total daily calorie intake.

126. Consume Less calories in Liquid Form

We seldom realize but we consume a great amount of calories in liquid form too. Juices, soda, sweetened tea or coffee and similar items add a lot of calories to our diet. Keeping a watch on the number of calories consumed in liquid form is important for limiting calorie intake.

127. Slow Cooker Meals are Good

The longer you take to cook a meal on slow flame the better is the result in terms of health. Slow cooked meals are easy to digest and give better results.

128. Schedule Cheat Meals

Having great self-control is great when it comes to a diet. However, you should schedule cheat meals once in a while so that you don't get tempted at the first sight of inviting food. Planning keeps you in the driver's seat.

129. Try to Take all the Sugar from Fruits

Refined and processed sugars not only add too many calories to your diet but they are also difficult to process. The insulin resistance increases with high intake of sugar in such forms. You should try to take your quota of sugar from naturally sweet products like fruits, resins and other such items. They offer simple forms of sugar that are easily dissolvable and don't cause problems.

130. Stand Up More Than You Sit

This is a **no-brainer**. When the focus is on burning more calories and being physically active, standing wins the race from sitting hands down. It will keep your metabolism running and burn more calories.

Chapter 9: Diet Tips

131. Eat Lots of Water-Rich Foods

Water-rich foods make you feel full pretty quick. You consume less calories and they also help in detoxification of the system.

132. Veggies Should Be the Biggest Part of a Meal

Veggies are undeniably the best food to lose weight. They are full of fiber and vital nutrients. They give you less fat and calories. You must bulk up your meal with veggies.

133. Cereals are Best for Breakfast

Cereals provide the best nutrition for breakfast. They are full of fiber and protein. You feel fuller and satiated for longer. You must include them in your breakfast.

134. Hot Sauce, Salsa and Cajun Seasoning

These are low caloric additives to food. They increase the flavor of the food but also make you feel fuller and more satiated at a much faster pace. You should include them in your diet.

135. Eat Fruits in Place of Fruit Juice

Fruit juices are extracted from fruits only yet fruits are a much better choice. Fruits contain fiber that is important for your digestive system and you can drink more fruits than you can eat. Eating fruits is comparatively slow and tedious and hence you'll feel satiated fast.

136. Chose Lighter Milk

Milk gives you protein and it is good for health but the higher the fat content the more difficult weight loss will be. Lower the fat content of your milk by one level. You should ultimately aim for skimmed milk that has the lowest calories but equal amount of protein and calcium.

137. Snack on Nuts

Nuts are a healthy choice when it comes to snacking. They help in reduce hunger pangs without giving you too many calories. They are full of nutritious fibers and vitamins too.

138. Avoid Junk Food

This point has been repeated several times yet it can't be stressed enough. If weight loss is your target then junk food should be a no-go at all costs. It adds weight and calories through unhealthy fats, refined sugars and salts.

139. Eat Lots of Blueberries

Recent studies have found that blueberries influence genes that regulate fat burning and storage. They are also very effective in regulating your blood sugar and triglyceride levels. You should eat them a lot.

140. Eat Lots of Stone Fruits

Stone fruits like plums, peaches and cherries are rich in pectin and fiber. Both these things help in burning fat faster as they are natural fat burners. They also help in improving your metabolism.

141. Eat Fresh Food

Processed meal can never take the place of fresh food. It is healthy, nutritious and low on calories. You have complete control of the calories you want to eat. Try to cook fresh food whenever possible.

142. Begin Your Day with Fiber

Fiber is the best filler you can have in your diet. It makes you feel fuller and also aids your digestion. You should begin your day with fiber.

143. Spice Up Your Food

Herbs and spices don't add calories to your food but have several anti-inflammatory advantages. They make your food tasty and also bring satiety faster.

144. Drink Green Tea

Green tea is a refreshing beverage. You can drink green tea without the guilt of consuming calories and it even helps in burning calories.

145. Eat Whole Grain Foods

Whole grain foods like brown rice, whole oats, unhulled barley have lots of fiber. They improve the digestive system and aid weight loss.

146. Limit Refined carbohydrates

Refined carbs are low in fiber and get digested fast. They give you an instant burst of energy and spike your blood sugar levels. Eating too much refined carbs will lead to faster weight gain and must be avoided.

147. Add Eggs to Your Diet

Eggs are the white gold for diet. They are rich in protein and make you feel fuller for much longer. Eating egg white will decrease your calorie intake and make you feel fuller. You must make it an essential part of your weight loss diet.

148. Probiotics

Probiotics are good for a healthy gut. They promote the production of good bacteria in your digestive system and keep you healthy.

149. Bring Healthy Fats to Your Diet

Omega-3 fatty acid rich healthy fats in form of fish and nuts are great for your weight loss. They promote health and fulfill your fat needs without compromising on health. You must add them to your diet.

150. Eat Lean Meats

Meat is an essential part of our diet. However, it is also full of fat that leads to weight gain. You should consider lean meats for faster weight loss. Skinless chicken, turkey, pork chops are good options for you.

151. Fish is the Best

Coldwater fish like salmon, mackerel, and sardines are rich in Omega-3 fatty acids and antioxidants. They provide great health benefits without adding much weight. They should be an ideal part of weight loss diet plan.

152. Avoid Inflammatory Foods

Refined carbohydrates, fried food, soda, red meat and processed meat and margarine can cause inflammation. This will ultimately lead to weight gain. You must avoid these foods to stay healthy and lean.

153. Switch from White Potato to Sweet Potato

White potatoes are a rich source of carbohydrates. They provide a lot of calories. Whereas, sweet potatoes have relatively low calories content. If you are trying to lose weight then sweet potatoes will be the best for you.

154. Lemons are Good

This citrus fruit is good for you. They act as mild diuretic and also keep your metabolism running. Drinking lemon juice can be a healthy addition to your weight loss plan.

155. Curb Your Sugar Cravings

Refined sugar in any form is bad for you as our body can't process it naturally. Our liver processes it as glycogen as stores it as fat. Eating one piece of anything sweet will make you long for more. It adds weight and calories. You must avoid it as much as possible.

156. Don't Eat Till Your Heart's Content

Our brain needs up to 20 minutes after you have eaten the last morsel of food to realize that you're full. So, when you feel that you've eaten 80% of your meal you've consumed you must stop. Do not wait for your brain to signal you to stop as by that time you'd have overeaten a lot.

157. Eat Good Carbs

All carbs are not bad as they are the main source of energy. However, you must avoid refined carbs and stress on getting carbs from whole grains. barley, whole wheat, beans and other such things give you good carbs.

158. Swap Unhealthy Food

There are times when eating out cannot be avoided. In such cases, insist on eating food items that are healthy. Avoid fried items or highly processed food products.

159. Switch From Simple Carbs to Complex Carbs

A rose by any name might be true for flowers but it isn't true to carbs. Simple carbs only add calories whereas complex carbs help you in losing weight. Our body needs time to digest them and hence your calorie intake reduces.

160. Go Low on Sodium

High sodium intake leads to greater water retention. It improves the taste of food and encourages overeating. Studies have also shown that salt makes the fat cells larger adding to weight gain.

Chapter 10: Foods That Help in Weight Loss

Seeds

161. Quinoa

Quinoa is rich in protein and fiber and accelerates weight loss. Protein takes longer to break down and consumes more energy in the process. This burns more calories for you.

162. Flax Seeds

Flax seeds are rich in fiber and improve your digestion. It makes you feel full and the fiber takes long to digest. This keeps your stomach engaged. In turn, you consume less calories.

163. Hemp Seeds

Hemp seeds are a rich source of protein, fiber and Omega-3 fatty acids. They help you greatly in weight loss. The improve your digestion and keep you feeling full for very long.

164. Chia Seeds

Chia seeds are also very rich in fiber. Two tablespoons of chia seeds contain almost 10 grams of fiber. They improve digestion and keep you satiated.

165. Farro

Farro has a very high amount of fiber. It aids digestion and helps in weight loss. It has almost twice the amount of fiber found in quinoa and three times the amount of fiber found in rice.

166. Kamut

Kamut is rich in protein and other essential nutrients. It also lowers the blood glucose levels in your body. It is an excellent weight loss food.

167. Oats

Oats take a lot of time to get digested and hence they are good for weight loss. They have a high amount of fiber and help in keeping your blood sugar levels low.

168. Sauerkraut

Sauerkraut is a pro-bacteria food and it helps in long-term weight loss efforts. This fermented food is good for your gut and keeps you healthy.

169. Brown Rice

Brown rice is great for burning fat and it has good amount of fiber. This is a low energy density food that keeps your metabolism running.

170. Whole Wheat

Whole wheat is best if you are trying to bring down belly fat. It has good amount of fiber and healthy carbohydrates.

Vegetables

171. Celery

Celery has a good reputation as a diet food. It has very low calorie content and very high nutritional value. It detoxifies your body.

172. Asparagus

Asparagus is low in fat and calories and also contains soluble and insoluble fiber. It keeps you satiated and helps in losing weight. It is also anti-inflammatory.

173. Spinach

Spinach is full of antioxidants and low on calories. It helps in fighting inflammation and doesn't add anything to your weight. It is a great addition to a weight loss diet.

174. Collard Greens

Collard Greens are known as the fat fighters. They are rich in beta-carotene and Vitamin C and fiber too. They add no calorie to your food and offer vital benefits.

175. Brussels Sprouts

Brussels sprouts are low in calorie and the high in fiber. They help digestion and also lower cholesterol levels.

176. Broccoli

Broccoli is full of nutrients and minerals. It is full of fiber and has low energy density. It has 90 percent water and the high fiber content helps you in losing weight.

178. Cabbage

Cabbage is full of insoluble fiber and helps you in quickly losing a few pounds. It drastically limits your calorie intake.

179. Green Beans

Green Beans are full of fiber and quickly give a feeling of fullness. They limit your food intake by bringing satiety. They are very effective for weight loss.

180. Zucchini

Zucchini is one of the best sources of dietary fiber and helps in keeping your body in good shape in the long run. It has excellent anti-inflammatory properties too.

181. Cauliflower

Cauliflower is a non-starchy food which you can eat in large quantities without worrying about weight. It helps you in your weight loss efforts.

182. Carrots

Carrots are low in calories and high in fiber. They fill up your stomach and their nutrients help in weight loss.

183. Cayenne Pepper

Cayenne pepper improves your metabolism and provides nutrients. Due to its spicy nature it helps in burning calories too.

184. Mushrooms

Mushrooms are great for weight loss. They are rich in fiber and protein. They offer low calorie count. You can bring mushrooms to your diet for effective weight loss.

185. Artichoke

Artichoke increases the bile production in your liver and helps in getting rid of bad cholesterol. It is rich in dietary fiber and also lowers the blood glucose levels. It is a great addition to the weight loss diet.

186. Eggplant

Eggplant is a great food for weight loss. It is a nutrient rich and has very few calories and carbohydrates. One cup of eggplant only contains 8 grams of carbohydrates.

187. Okra

The fiber in okra acts as the fuel for gut bacteria. It helps in the metabolism of fat. The fiber in okra also helps in the transportation of fat-soluble toxins which is great for your health. It regulates your blood sugar and helps in weight loss.

188. Pumpkin

Pumpkin is low in calories and has high dietary fiber content. One cup of pumpkin only contains 40 calories but 8 grams of fiber. It keeps your blood sugar level under control and helps in weight loss.

189. Garlic

Garlic has great anti-inflammatory properties and increases the metabolism rate in the body. It decreases the fat levels in the blood and improves the functioning of liver. In addition to these, garlic is also an appetite suppressant.

190. Ginger

Ginger has excellent health properties and it is known around the world for its antioxidant values. It assists your digestive system and promotes weight loss.

Berries

191. Blueberries

Blueberries influence the fat-burning genes in the body. They are especially helpful in burning abdominal fat and lowering your cholesterol levels. You should consume them on regular basis.

192. Blackberries

Blackberries are an excellent source of fiber and have very few calories. They fill you up faster without adding many calories. They can be a part of your weight loss diet.

193. Raspberries

Raspberries are full of fiber and water. They contain no fat and provide very few calories. You can eat them instead of sweets and promote weight loss. The high fiber content in them takes very long to get digested and they keep your stomach full.

194. Strawberries

Strawberries are a rich source of vitamins, minerals, antioxidants, and fiber. They provide very few calories as a cup of strawberries will only give you 49 calories. You can make them a part of your weight loss diet.

195. Tart Cherries

Tart cherries are rich in fiber and provide anti-inflammatory benefits. They help in filling up your stomach without adding too many calories. They can become a part of ideal weight loss diet.

Fruits

196. Grapefruit

Grapefruit can help you in filling you up and reduce your appetite. You can drink a glass of grapefruit juice or eat half of the grapefruit before meals and you'll eat less food. It will reduce your calorie intake.

197. Watermelon

Watermelon in 92 percent water and has 2 grams of fiber per one cup serving. It fills you up and reduces your appetite. It flushes out toxins from your body and also improves your digestive system.

198. Peach

It is low in calories and completely fat-free. It is also a good source of vitamins. It provides natural sugar that's easily usable. It helps in burning extra fat deposits in the body.

199. Avocados

Avocados are the best for your low-calorie diet. 50 grams of avocados only contain 80 calories. They lower your cholesterol levels and reduce your hunger pangs. They are great for weight loss

200. Pomegranates

Pomegranates are rich in antioxidants and are good for your health. They also suppress your appetite and help you in following a calorie deficient diet. They can be a great addition to your weight loss diet.

Healthy Fats

Fish

201. Mackerel

Mackerel is an oily fish that is low on calories and rich in Omega-3 fatty acids. The polyunsaturated fat in this fish helps in reducing cholesterol levels and inflammation. It is a great addition to a weight loss diet.

202. Sardines

Sardines are loaded with proteins and regulate your blood sugar levels. they make you feel fuller very quickly and also stimulates your metabolism. They have antioxidant properties and help in weight loss.

203. Wild Salmon

Wild salmon is a power food. It is rich in proteins and low in calories. 3 ounces of salmon only carries 155 calories but 22 grams of protein. It has 7 grams of fat but most of it is very healthy for you. This fish has ample health benefits to include in all kinds of diets.

204. Trout

Trout is also low in calories and high in protein. A cup of trout has 179 calories and 39 grams of protein. It is also rich in Omega-3 fatty acids and other nutrients. It is a good choice for weight loss diet.

205. Shrimps

Shrimps are protein packed and have very low calories. They offer other health benefits too like vitamins and minerals. They boost your energy levels and help in losing weight.

Meat

206. Chicken

It is a lean meat that should be a part of your weight loss diet. It is full of protein along with calcium and phosphorous. It boosts satiety and you can easily lose weight with chicken on your diet.

207. Turkey

It is even leaner than chicken and has much better proportion of saturated and unsaturated fats. It is also high in protein content. It gives you less calories and fat percentage. 3 ounces of turkey only has 170 calories and 7 grams of fat.

208. Lamb

Leaner portions of lamb can be added to a weight loss diet as they contain less calories. However, visible fat should be trimmed and only the leaner portions should be consumed.

209. Pork Chops

Pork chops can be a part of your balanced diet as they provide beneficial nutrients and are low in calories and fat. However, you must avoid overeating them and restrict your diet to 3 ounces of pork chops.

210. Lean Beef

It is rich in protein and low in calories. It is loaded with antioxidants and minerals. You get less calories and fat from lean beef and get great benefits. You can include lean beef in your diet but must ensure that it is lean ground beef.

Vegetables

211. Lentils

They make up for excellent weight loss food. They have high fiber content and low-fat protein. The fiber helps in losing weight and protein helps in muscle building. They reduce your craving for food and also stabilize your blood sugar levels.

212. Kidney Beans

They are protein rich and induce satiety. They have low carbohydrate and fat content and help in reducing your craving for food for very long.

213. Garbanzo Beans

They have very high fiber content and no sugar at all. You get very few calories on eating these beans and they are an excellent addition to weight loss diet.

Nuts

214. Macadamia Nuts

These nuts can be eaten in a number of ways and offer great health benefits. They contain healthy fats and are very good for your heart. Besides, they also make you feel fuller and reduce your craving for food. You can snack on them when hungry.

215. Pistachios

Pistachios have high fiber and protein content and make you feel satisfied and reduce your craving for food. They are a healthy snack and offer great health benefits. However, you must avoid eating too much of them.

216. Almonds

Almonds have a lot of health benefits. They contain monounsaturated fats that prevent overeating. The dietary fiber in almonds also makes you feel fuller. You can snack on them when feeling hungry.

217. Walnuts

Studies have found that eating walnuts accelerates fat burning. It lowers bad cholesterol in your body and promotes the production of good cholesterol. They should be a part of your weight loss diet.

218. Peanuts

Studies show that the monounsaturated fats in peanuts promote weight loss and prevent heart diseases.

219. Pine Nuts

Pine nuts release fatty acids that suppress appetite. If you are following a weight loss diet and are having problems in calorie restriction then these nuts can provide the perfect solution.

220. Dark Chocolate

Dark Chocolate can help you in reducing weight. It helps in stabilizing blood sugar levels, controlling appetite and reducing craving. If you are on a weight loss diet then this indulgence can help you.

Chapter 11: Important Things to Follow

221. Fix Time for Having Meals

This will regulate your craving for food. After some time your body would stop craving food at odd times.

222. Don't Force Food

Learn to say no when it comes to food. If you aren't feeling very hungry then don't eat.

223. Always Eat Fresh and Warm Food

This rule will help in removing most of the food temptations which do not pass on this rule. You'll get better and healthier food.

224. Eat at a Peaceful Place

Eating is an important activity for your body. Eat at a peaceful place that helps in generating positive energy.

225. Be Cheerful

Stress and anxiety are big factors that contribute to weight gain. You can lose weight faster by remaining happy and positive.

226. Eat Quietly

Talking while eating or watching television may lead to excessive eating as your attention is elsewhere. You must avoid it.

227. Don't Drink Much Water While Eating

Drinking too much water while eating is bad for your digestion. It weakens the food canal and you aren't able to process the food properly.

228. Chew Your Food Well

Chewing is an important part of eating. Chewing the food properly makes it easier to digest. It also consumes more time and you feel full even with less food.

229. Don't Eat Immediately After a Stressful Workout

Let the temperature of your body get back to normal otherwise there will be problems in digesting the food properly.

230. Don't Eat in a Hurry

Always eat food slowly as it gives you proper time to chew and you can easily avoid overeating.

231. Maintain a Time Gap Between Meals

Always keep a specific time gap between meals. This will help you in avoiding overeating or mindless eating. The gap should be minimum three hours and up to 5 hours.

232. Drink Water in the Morning

Water is a magical drink. It keeps your digestive system healthy and flushes out toxins from your system. Every morning drink water on empty stomach. This will keep you healthy.

233. Reduce the Consumption of Fatty Products

Fat accumulates faster and it is very difficult to burn. Avoiding foods that lead to fat accumulation is the best. Make it a habit to eat low fat foods.

234. Make Up Your Mind Before Eating

Before you sit for meal decide in advance the thing you want to eat. Don't decide it by looking at the contents in the fridge. This habit leads to overeating.

235. Treat Temptations Carefully

You should not curb your temptations all the time. If you are feeling like eating something then eat it in controlled quantity. This will stop your mind from revolting.

236. Do Exercise Regularly

No diet can take the place of exercise. It keeps you fresh and healthy and you are able to burn fat faster and efficiently.

237. Don't Try to Get Instant Results

The desire for instant results is very strong. However, it is unsustainable. Even if you are able to lose weight it will have negative impact on your health and your body will not be able to adjust to the change. Maintaining that weight is nearly impossible as you return to your normal routine. Go for a steady and sustainable weight loss regimen.

238. Focus on Consuming Less Calories

Weight loss diet is primarily about consuming less calories and more fiber. Your goal should always be that. If your calorie intake increases your weight will also go down.

239. Burn More Calories

You must try to burn more calories than you consume. It is very simple math. If you are not burning more than you are consuming then your weight will not go down.

240. Don't Indulge in Binge Eating

This is simply unhealthy and must be avoided at all costs. It will nullify all your efforts.

Eating Out

241. Check the Menus Online

While eating out it gets difficult to control the amount of calories. Prepare in advance and if possible check the menu online so that you already have the options in mind. Deciding on the spot can force you to make impulsive decisions.

242. Grilled, Baked, Boiled

Look for grilled, baked and boiled items as they are most likely to have the least calories and fats.

243. Munch Some Nuts Beforehand

Eating a few nuts will suppress your appetite and you'll consume a few less calories than normal.

244. Begin with Fiber-Rich Items

Salads are the best to start your meal outside. They make you feel full quite early and cause the least damage.

245. Sauces and Dressings are Good

Sauces and dressings not only spice up the food but also induce satiety.

246. Go for Baked in Place of Fries

Fried food items are very rich in fats and calories. It will rupture your weight loss diet plan. Go for baked items as they are healthy.

247. Prefer Greens

Greens are always healthy irrespective of the place. Whenever possible choose the greens for your meals.

248. Be Careful with Wine

Red wine is good in controlled quantities but excess is bad for everything. Try to order glasses of wine instead of a full bottle.

249. Don't Order Too Much

Ordering more food puts a burden to finish. Order in small quantities so that you don't have to force feed yourself.

250. Be Careful with Desserts

Sweets are good but they add too many calories. Try to limit your dessert intake. If possible share it with your partner(s).

Wrapping-up

Thanks for making it through to the end of this book, let's hope it was informative and able to provide you with all of the tools you need to achieve your goals whatever they may be.

Losing weight requires a lot of effort and self-control. Quick solutions don't work. It is one of the biggest reasons that even after getting expensive fat reduction surgeries the weight comes back.

This book helps you in reducing your weight through simple and effective diet control. It guides and motivates you to cut your calorie intake and burn more calories. It stresses on the sustainable model for weight loss.

You do not need expensive equipment or costly diet supplements to do this. You can cut down your weight by living a simple life through modest means. All you need is self-control, discipline, and planning.

You will have to restrict yourself some time and sacrifice your craving for food at times. The methods and tricks given in the book will help you all through your journey.

It is a complete guide for effective weight loss. It doesn't offer quick fixes but gives you a detailed path to lose weight in the long run. The biggest advantage of the ways given in the book is that it will help you in managing that weight easily and you wouldn't get overweight again very soon.

Finally, if you found this book useful in any way, a review on Amazon is always appreciated!

MEAL PREP GUIDE

TIME MANAGEMENT FOR THE KITCHEN

The Ultimate Guide to Achieving Your Weight Loss Goals

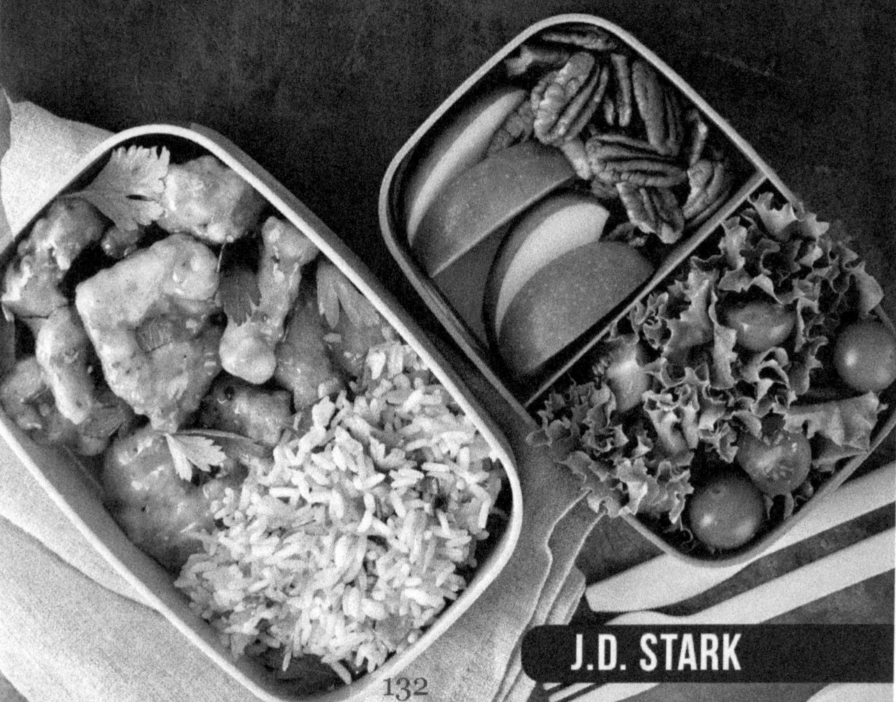

J.D. STARK

Meal Prep Guide:

Time Management for the Kitchen

By J.D. Stark
jd-stark.com

Table of Contents

interim quality. Trademarks that mentioned are done without written consent and can in no way be considered an endorsement from the trademark holder.

Introduction

Congratulations on downloading the *Meal Prep Guide: Time Management for the Kitchen* and thank you for doing so.

There are many articles and websites that commend the virtues of meal prepping. Calling it out as the simplest method to eat healthier, and control portions. However, it seems, that they leave out the essential building block of what meal prepping is, at its heart. It is a tool for time management.

By using a larger block of time on a weekend, usually a Sunday, you are essentially saving time during the week, no hasty breakfasts, no fast food lunches, no last-minute dinners while rushing through evening activities.

Meal prepping will keep your daily schedule on track without cutting corners. Utilizing the tools in this guide will allow you maximize your free time while ensuring your meals are full of flavor, variety and most of all flexibility.

There are plenty of books on this subject on the market, thanks again for choosing this one! Every effort was made to ensure it is full of as much useful information as possible; so please enjoy!

Chapter 1: What is Meal Prep?

Boiled down, meal prepping is simply the mastery of making leftovers. It really is just that simple. You're going to make several large dishes that are compatible with each other and then mix and match them throughout the week.

Your prepping will start with a plan – this in no way needs to be a long, exhaustive production. I feel it's always best to use the KISS method (keep it simple stupid). Don't plan a long drawn out menu that will take 8 hours in the kitchen too cook, not only will you have a mountain of dishes to clean, but you will become discouraged from meal prepping in the future because it took up an entire day.

So, let's begin, grab a pen/pencil and a pad of paper, and think about what you have planned for the upcoming week. If you work out often, you're going to want to ensure that you will have not only enough protein but also easy and portable snacks. If you know that you'll be on the road or running around shuttling the family from one spot to another, you'll need to have quick snacks and meals essentials that don't take a lot of time to throw together.

This is an excellent opportunity to grab that Costco or Sam's Club Membership, while you're browsing for sale mega packs of chicken breasts, you'll be able to take advantage of all those free samples, and let's be honest a trip through Costco trying samples is a meal in itself.

The simplest way to break down your list/plan will be to divide it into sections Protein, Vegetables, Fats, Carbs, and Other (by which I mean dessert, because chocolate, is always on the menu). When you're putting together your plate, you'll want to ensure you have 1 protein, 1 vegetable, and 1 healthy carb.

For Example:

- Carbs: Quinoa, rice, beans/lentils, chickpeas, potatoes (skin on), steel-cut oats
- Protein: Chicken, turkey, lean beef, bison, salmon, eggs, tofu, Greek yogurt
- Veggies: Asparagus, broccoli, cauliflower, green beans, Brussels sprouts, kale, spinach, beets, squash (every kind), zucchini
- Fats: Avocado, olive oil, olives, coconut oil
- Snacks: Apples, berries, almonds, dark chocolate, pumpkin seeds, peanuts

The above is in no way a comprehensive list, but it gives you some good places to start and allows a large amount of mix and match options. Now when it comes to snacks, a word of warning: *nuts are not free food*, if you're looking to lose weight. They pack a lot of calories into a small package which is very easy to overeat without noticing.

Just remember; meal prep means something different to every situation. Whether you are making enough food for 12 hours or 12 weeks; it's the same logic – saving time. The following chapters will provide you with the path to your new way of eating!

Chapter 2: The Basics

Now to the Essentials:

You're going to need plastic wrap, tin foil, wax paper, and lots food storage containers. The best ones are clear, so when they're stacked in the fridge; you can tell what the contents are without any guesswork. Mason jars are also great and a lot of fun for salads; you can layer different colored vegetables in them and then just add dressing and shake, it doesn't get much easier than that, plus, it's just so darn fancy.

Roasted vegetables are your friend; not only are they easy to make in bulk, but you can also roast them on the same pan with a little help from your friend 'tin foil', and they are often on sale in the frozen food section. So, if you break down 3 or 4 different veggies for one week, you've got yourself covered.

Barbecued anything is good! This is especially true of chicken, and no one ever minds eating it more than once each week. A pan of roasted chicken breasts can be jazzed up with BBQ seasoning and lemon pepper. Just divide the two halves of the pan with tin foil, and you've just shaved 45 min. off your cooking time.

Talking about seasoning. This will be your savior; it's a quick and easy way to jazz up any meal. You can add it to meats, vegetables, and carbs. It requires very little effort and can take a 'blah' meal to a 'yum' meal in seconds. Garlic, lemon, rosemary, thyme, sage - all of them pack a flavor punch, so don't be afraid to experiment.

Make the protein your base. If there was a sale on fish or chicken, make 3 different flavors of that protein. You don't have to make tuna, salmon, chicken, and turkey all at once, that's just exhausting, it's much easier to make 1 protein and simply change up the spices so that it seems like you're getting 3 different items.

Bulk prep your carbs. Make a large pot of lentils, beans or quinoa; then you can either divide it into 2 or 3 different flavors with your herbs and spices or space it out over your containers and add a sauce to finish it off.

Now another note of caution. Don't over prep. While you certainly don't want to run out of meals or short yourself on portions; you don't want to make so much food that you end up throwing it away. Not only is it wastefully expensive, but it's also eating into your free time since you had to cook all of the extras. Look at a reasonable portion size for you. If you know you'll eat 1 chicken breast per meal, then prep enough chicken breast for each meal you intend to have it for. Make 10, not 15.

Think about variety and options, such as boiled eggs; they are quick, easy and versatile. Add in precut raw veggies for snacking, mixing it up by including proportioned servings of cottage cheese or cut pieces of fruit, like apples along with the small premeasured packets of peanut or almond butter. These all make great go-to snacks either for between meetings at work, for the kids on the way to soccer practice or if you're just feeling 'pinchy' between meals.

Dessert - everyone's favorite part of the day. Why deny yourself? When you proportion out your servings, there are no fears that you'll demolish an entire box of Oreos. While 100 calorie packs are perfectly nice, but why get a little adventurous, you're already in the kitchen, how about a quick blender fruit puree, portioned out into a Tupperware container, for a cool treat later; or peanut/almond butter and thinly sliced fruit on graham crackers, you can slide them in a baggie and keep them in the fridge, perfect for a late night snack or if you're in an on the go rush; you can even get a little wild and sprinkle the peanut/almond butter with mini dark chocolate chips.

Now that you have the basics, it's time to start the process. Each of the following recipes will provide you with the servings and method of storage listed before the rest of the information. This is a unique feature that will allow you to plan ahead with your menu. You can increase the amounts suggested to fit your household. Use what you need and freeze the rest.

It is always good to have a written inventory, but not essential. You will soon know what works best for you.

Get Down to Basics

These are several of the many ways you can get down to basics and always be prepared:

Eggs

The Meal Prep Method: You can hard-boil the eggs to last for a week and store them in the refrigerator. Leave the shells on and in the original carton, but remember to mark the carton with the date and time. You can also use them in sandwiches or with a salad – anytime!

Extra Tip: The reason to refrain from peeling the eggs - lies in the fact they can absorb and create smells and mix flavors. You don't want that to happen - so be sure the container used is airtight. Just place the whole carton into a zip-lock type bag for safe and easy access.

Chicken

The Meal-Prep Method: Program the oven temperature to 350°F. Coat your meat in a tablespoon or two of oil and apply the seasonings. Bake approximately 30 minutes.

For a change of pace, season half your chicken one way and use a different set of flavorings for the other half. Once baked, let it cool slightly, then divide three-ounce cuts into multiple airtight containers. Just place an aluminum foil liner between the two flavors.

Since cooked chicken can't quite last the full week in the fridge, cut up anything you'll use after day three (at the latest) and place in individual freezer bags. Then freeze until it's time to eat.

Extra Tip: Chicken breasts may be the leanest, but for meal-prep purposes, thighs may be a better bet. Their slightly higher fat content means they won't become as dry in the fridge, plus they're cheaper!

Remember that it's safest to reheat chicken only once, so warm up only the amount you plan to eat. Chicken is best reheated the way it was cooked, so spread the pieces on a cookie sheet. Set the oven setting to 450°F. Cover with aluminum foil. Bake for about 10 minutes.

Ground Meats

The Meal Prep Method: Warm up a skillet, then add the meat, cooking it until it's evenly browned. Once cooled, pack three-ounce portions into several airtight containers. Like chicken, the ground meat won't last longer than three days in the fridge, so pack anything you'll use after day three into freezer bags, squeezing out as much air as possible before sealing and freezing. Use the meat for pasta sauce, tacos, and casseroles. Be creative. Only you know what your family likes!

Extra Tip: Ground meat lasts longer cooked than raw, so be sure to remove it from the store packaging and cook it as soon as possible. Make your frozen ground meat last longer by thawing it in the fridge rather than a microwave. Doing so will keep the meat safe to use for an additional day or two.

Grains

Oatmeal

The Meal-Prep Method: Have breakfast half-ready all week long by simmering a pinch of salt, one and a half cups of steel-cut oats, and four cups of water for three minutes before turning off the heat. Once the mixture comes down to room temperature, place the oatmeal in an airtight container. You should get about five servings.

Extra Tip: Save even more time in the morning by packing the oatmeal into five individual containers and mix with your favorite add-ins. Before heading out the door, add a splash of water or milk to one jar, and reheat in the microwave—or just eat cold for the easiest overnight oats ever!

Pasta

The Meal-Prep Method: Boil 10 ounces of pasta according to package instructions, but take it off the stove when it's just shy of al dente; you'll want it slightly undercooked so that it's not mushy when you reheat it during the week. Drain the pasta in a colander using cold tap water to stop the cooking process. Toss the pasta in a splash of olive oil and place it into a tightly sealed container. You should have about (five) one-cup servings.

Bonus Tip: Make your pasta last longer by storing it separately from sauces and add-ins. For a fast reheating option, prepare a pot of boiling water. Put your chosen pasta in a metal strainer and dip it into the boiling water for about thirty seconds, or until it's warmed through - but not soggy.

Quinoa

The Meal-Prep Method: Rinse one cup of quinoa, then place it in a pot with two cups of water along with about 1/8 teaspoon of salt. Once it boils, add a lid to the pot and lower the heat. Let it cook slowly (15 min.) until the liquid is gone. Let it sit for five minutes before fluffing with a fork. Cool, then store in airtight containers. You should get about (six) half-cup servings.

Extra Tip: Make quinoa last longer and taste even better by reheating it on the stovetop. Add about two tablespoons of water for every cup of quinoa, plus a teaspoon of olive oil. Heat it in a pot for 10 minutes or until it's warmed through and fluffy.

Brown Rice

The Meal-Prep Method: Rinse one cup of short-grain brown rice in cold water. Add the rice to one and a half cups of boiling water and cook for about 30 minutes, covered. Let it sit for another 10 minutes before opening and fluffing with a fork. Cool, then store in shallow, airtight containers. You should get about (five) half-cup servings.

Extra Tip: Cooked brown rice will keep for about five days in the fridge. To make it taste fresher, reheat only the portion you need for a given meal during the week. For speedy reheating, place the rice in a microwave-safe dish, and sprinkle some water over the top. Cover the dish with a wet paper towel. Nuke on high heat until the rice is back to its steamy.

Fruit Prep

Apples

The Meal-Prep Method: Apples are one of the lowest-maintenance fruits out there. Leave them whole and refrigerated in the crisper drawer to keep them fresh for up to four weeks. If you must slice or chop them, place the pieces in a glass container filled with cold water to prevent oxidization and browning.

Extra Tip: Place a damp paper towel over whole apples in the fridge—the moisture helps them stay fresh longer. Alternatively, put them in sealed plastic bags and keep them separate from other products to prevent ethylene gas from releasing and causing spoilage.

Bananas

The Meal-Prep Method: Even ripe bananas can last all week with a few simple tricks. Take them out of any plastic bags as soon as possible and separate each banana from the bunch. Wrap each banana's stem in a bit of plastic wrap, and place in the fridge. The wrap will prevent the ripening and browning agents from spreading to the rest of the banana too quickly, and the refrigeration will keep the fruit firm.

Bonus Tip: Make bananas last even longer by peeling and cutting them into one-inch chunks, then placing them on parchment paper and freezing. Once frozen, put them in freezer bags and keep for up to four months to throw into baked goods, smoothies, or one ingredient ice cream.

Berries

Meal-Prep Method: Are you surprised to see berries on this list? While the jewel-colored fruits are notorious for spoiling easily, there is an easy way to keep them fresh all week. Add one cup of vinegar to three cups of water in a large bowl, and soak the berries in the mixture for about five minutes. Drain the berries and pat them until they're as dry as you can get them. Place them in an airtight container that's been lined with paper towels and crack the lid open to keep letting moisture escape.

Bonus Tip: Keep in mind that despite this method, certain berries still hold up better than others. Choose strawberries and blueberries over blackberries or raspberries, and try to keep them in a single layer rather than piling them on top of each other to prevent bruising.

Grapes

The Meal-Prep Method: Grapes can last up to two to three weeks when stored properly. Line an open container with a paper towel and place the grapes on top. The towel will help draw out any extra moisture from the fruit and keep out bacteria or mold growth. Keep the grapes in the coldest part of your fridge.

Bonus Tip: For longest-lasting results, don't rinse the grapes until just before you're ready to eat them. Even if you do happen to wash them beforehand, though, they can still keep for up to a week if refrigerated.

Now, it's time to move on to the meal plans!

Chapter 3 – Breakfasts

Here is a ton of suggestions for at least one weeks' worth of prepped breakfasts. You can make as much using these mixtures as you wish.

Almond & Berry Breakfast Quinoa

Servings: 4
Method of Storage: Refrigerator

This is what you'll need:

- 2 c. almond milk – regular
- 1 c. quinoa
- ¼ t. ground cardamom
- ½ t. ground cinnamon
- 2 tbsp. maple syrup
- 4. c. mixed berries
- 4 tbsp. sliced almonds

Instructions
1. Combine the milk, quinoa, cardamom, and cinnamon in a medium saucepan. After the mixture starts boiling, just lower the heat setting to low and simmer slowly for about 15 minutes.
2. Cool, stir in the syrup, and divide into the containers (4).
3. Use this as a guideline:
   a. ¾ c. cooked quinoa
   b. 1 c. fruit
   c. 1 tbsp. sliced almonds

Apple Raisin Instant Oatmeal

Servings: 1
Method of Storage: Room temperature

This is what you'll need:

- 1/3 c. chopped dried apples
- ½ cup oats
- ¼ c. raisins
- ¼ t. ground cinnamon
- Pinch – salt
- Optional to Taste: Pinch of sugar/substitute
- ½ c. boiling water

Instructions
1. For one serving, mix all of the fixings in a canning jar (pint sized) or a container with a tight-fitting lid. Store in the cabinet until ready to use.
2. Prepare the Oats: Pour in the water, stir, and let rest for five minutes.
3. Then, dive in!

Avocado & Eggs

Servings: 4
Method of Storage: Refrigerator

This is what you'll need:

- 1 c. water
- ½ c. brown rice
- 2 tbsp. olive oil
- ¼ t. crushed red pepper flakes – optional
- 2 minced garlic cloves
- 4 c. chopped kale
- ¼ c. freshly grated Parmesan
- 1 avocado

Instructions
1. Cut the avocado in half, de-seed, peel, and slice.
2. Prepare the rice with the water. Let it rest.
3. Add the eggs to a saucepan with water covering them with at least one inch. Let it boil for one minute. Cover and remove from the burner (8-10 min.). Drain, cool, peel, and cut into halves.
4. Warm up the oil in a skillet (med-hi heat). Toss in the pepper flakes and garlic. Saute about one or two minutes. Fold in the kale and stir until wilted (5-6 min.). Shake in the parmesan.
5. Prepare the storage containers with equal portions for a quick breakfast.

Banana & Peanut Butter –Shake & Go Oats

Servings: 1
Method of Storage: Refrigerator

This is what you'll need:

- 1 t. chia seeds
- 1/3 – ½ c. rolled oats
- 1 tbsp. peanut butter
- ¼ t. cinnamon
- 1/8 t. vanilla extract
- ½ med. chopped banana
- ½ c. non-dairy soy/almond milk

Instructions
1. Combine the fixings in the order listed in a mason jar.
2. Shake well until mixed. Refrigerate overnight, pack, and go.

Breakfast Burritos

Servings: 4
Method of Storage: Freezer

This is what you'll need:

- 1 lb. ground turkey or shredded chicken
- 1 pkg. taco seasoning
- 1 can black beans, drained and rinsed/refried bean paste
- 1 c. chopped fresh Roma tomatoes
- 1 bag fresh spinach
- 5 eggs
- ¼ c. Half & Half
- To Taste: Pepper and salt
- 1 c. shredded cheddar cheese
- 1 pkg. of tortillas

Instructions
1. Brown the turkey. Once cooked, add the taco seasoning, tomatoes, and black beans. Stir over the medium heat setting and add the spinach until it just starts to wilt.
2. In a small bowl, add the eggs, Half & Half, salt, and pepper to taste.
3. Fold in the egg mixture to the spinach; cooking until scrambled. Blend in with the turkey mixture. Pour evenly over tortillas, add cheese and wrap up firmly.

You can wrap these in freezer paper and reheat later. Add a couple dollops of sour cream and maybe a little hot sauce for some extra zip.

Cheesy Quiche

Servings: 3
Method of Storage: Refrigerator

This is what you'll need:

- 6 eggs
- 1 c. Half & Half
- 2 tbsp. flour
- ¼ c. yellow onion (chopped)
- To Taste: Pepper and salt
- 8 ounces shredded Gruyere or sharp Cheddar cheese (or both)
- 1 package frozen chopped spinach
- 8 slices bacon (crispy and chopped)
- 1 Deep-dish unbaked pie shell

Instructions
1. Program the oven setting to 350ºF.
2. Whisk the Half & Half, eggs, and flour in a large mixing container. Next, add the rest of the fixings.
3. Scrape the batter into the unbaked deep pie crust.
4. Bake (45 min. – 1 hr.)

Egg Cups

The egg mixture here is only a base; you can add or subtract to taste.

This is what you'll need:

- Eggs – 6 eggs
- Sausage – Breakfast Style (loose)
- Spinach – 1 Bag (Fresh)
- Onion, Bell Pepper Mix (pre-cut or frozen)
- Brie – 1 Small Wheel Cut into 6 (½ inch) pieces (freeze the rest)
- Mushrooms – ½ c.
- Half and Half – ½ c.
- Salt & Pepper
- Butter

Instructions
1. Set the oven to 350°F. Butter muffin tin. Set aside.
2. Fry up loose breakfast sausage, add in onion - bell peppers, mushrooms, and spinach until soft. Spoon mixture evenly into 6 of the tins.
3. Whisk the eggs and Half & Half into a bowl, along with the salt and pepper to taste. Pour the egg mixture on top, leaving 1/4" from the top.
4. Press one piece of brie into each of the six tins.
5. Prepare in the oven approximately 20 minutes. Remove from oven. Use a knife to go around the edges. Enjoy!

Keep them in an airtight container or a plastic baggie; Dispose of after 5-6 days!

Lentil & Zucchini Breakfast Burritos

Servings: 6
Method of Storage: Freezer or Refrigerator

This is what you'll need:

- ½ c. chopped onion
- ½ tbsp. olive oil
- 1 chopped bell pepper
- 1 c. of each:
-    -Chopped zucchini
-    -Lentils – canned – drained and rinsed
- 6 eggs
- ¼ t. pepper
- ½ t. of each:
-    -Oregano
-    -Salt
- 2 c. shredded cheddar cheese
- 1 (12-inch) tortillas

Instructions
1. Warm up the oil using the medium heat setting on the stovetop. Toss in the onions and saute for five minutes. Then, add the peppers and zucchini. Continue to saute for about five more minutes.
2. In another container, whisk the eggs, with the oregano, pepper, and salt. Add the eggs to the pan of lentils and cook three to four minutes until the eggs are done.

Assemble the Burritos
1. Prepare ½ c. of the egg/veggie filling into each of the tortillas.
2. Sprinkle with 1/3 c. of cheese.
3. Roll and wrap in plastic wrap until ready to eat.

To Freeze and Thaw
1. After wrapping the burritos in the wrap; arrange them into a large Ziploc-type bag. If storing over one or two weeks; add a layer of foil.
2. You can store that overnight in the fridge or warm it up in the microwave (30 seconds per side).
3. Crisp them in a skillet or Foreman Grill before serving if you want them crispier.

Mexican Breakfast Taquitos

Servings: 20
Method of Storage: Freezer or Refrigerator – 1 week

This is what you'll need:

- 10 eggs
- 3 tbsp. olive oil – divided
- ½ finely cubed sweet potato
- 1 red/green sliced green pepper
- 1 sliced red onion
- 1 c. shredded cheddar cheese
- 1/3 c. chopped cilantro
- 20 corn tortillas

This is what you'll need for the turkey sausage:

- 1 lb. ground turkey
- 1 t. of each:
- -Paprika
- -Salt
- -Garlic powder
- -Dijon mustard
- 1 tbsp. fennel seeds
- ½ t. pepper

Instructions

1. Prepare the turkey sausage by combining all of the fixings into 20-thin and long sausages. Fry with one tablespoon of oil for 10-15 minutes using med-hi heat.
2. Add one tablespoon of oil to the pan on the same setting and add the potatoes with a pinch of salt. Saute about ten minutes. Stir in the onions and peppers; continuing to saute

another three to four minutes. Transfer to a container and paper towel the pan clean.
3. Whisk the eggs and warm up the oil in the pan. Continue over the med-hi setting and scramble the eggs (5-6 min.).
4. Prepare the oven to 350°F. Place the tortillas on two baking sheets. Add a bit of cheese, eggs, and turkey sausage along with some of the veggie mix and fresh cilantro. Roll into a mini wrap. Place each one (open side down) on the baking sheet.
5. Bake 10 minutes, remove and let cool. Wrap each one in plastic wrap
before freezing. They will be good for one week.
6. To reheat, just microwave one serving for 3 min. to 3 ½ seconds (3 at a time) if frozen; or 1-2 minutes if stored in the fridge.

Note: Freeze the sausages you are not using for use at a later time.

Quinoa & Banana Breakfast Bars

Servings: 9-12
Method of Storage: Air-tight Container for 3 days or Freeze

This is what you'll need:

- 1 c. of each:
- -Rinsed white quinoa
- -Rolled oats
- ½ t. of each:
- -Cinnamon
- -Baking powder
- Pinch of salt
- 2 tbsp. ground flaxseed
- 3 large mashed ripened bananas
- 3 tbsp. natural peanut/another nut butter
- 1 tbs. softened coconut oil
- 2 tbsp. pure maple syrup
- Optional: ¼- ½ c. unsweetened coconut or chopped dried fruit

- Also Needed: 9x9 baking dish

Instructions
1. Set the oven temperature to 350ºF.
2. Prepare the pan with coconut oil or non-stick cooking spray.
3. Combine the oats, baking powder, salt, cinnamon, and quinoa in a large mixing container.
4. Blend in the peanut butter, bananas, flax, syrup, and coconut oil. Stir until well incorporated. Sprinkle with the add-in fixings.
5. Let the batter rest about ten minutes for the seeds to absorb the juices.

6. Add the batter to the prepared pan and bake 25 minutes.
7. Cool for about 20 minutes before cutting into 9-12 squares.
8. Store in an air-tight container or freeze.

Sweet Potato Breakfast Bowls

Servings: 1
Method of Storage: Refrigerator

This is what you'll need:

- 2 tbsp. - 100% all-natural peanut butter – Kraft for ex.
- ½ c. mashed sweet potato

Instructions
1. Bake a small sweet potato and mash it in a bowl. Add the peanut butter, sliced strawberries, blueberries, and the rest of the desired toppings.
2. Store as many as you like in the fridge for easy access on those hurried mornings!

Yogurt & Fruit Cups

Servings: 4
Method of Storage: Refrigerator up to 3 days (life of the fruit varies)

This is what you'll need:

- 1 to 1 ¼ c. peeled & chopped fruit of choice:
  a. Oranges, berries, kiwi, mango, cherries, pineapple,
  b. Or (tossed with lemon juice)
- 1 ½ c. plain whole milk yogurt
- 4 (8 oz.) Mason jars

Instructions
1. Add several tablespoons of fruit in the bottom of the jars. Add the yogurt and more fruit.
2. Leave a bit of room on top if you want to add some other goodies such as muesli, granola, or nuts and seeds. Seal the jars.
3. Store the jars in the fridge up to three days, depending on the texture of the fruit.
4. Enjoy anytime by just adding your favorite toppings.

Zucchini & Banana Overnight Oats

Servings: 2
Method of Storage: Refrigerator 4-6 hrs. or overnight

This is what you'll need:

- 1 med. ripe banana
- 1 c. old-fashioned oats
- 1 1/3 c. unsweetened vanilla almond milk
- 1 c. grated zucchini
- ½ t. cinnamon
- Optional: 1 t. chia seeds

This is what you'll need for the toppings:

- Sliced banana
- Walnuts
- Almond butter
- Chocolate chips
- Maple syrup
- Coconut

Instructions
1. Arrange the banana in a medium dish and mash using a fork. Blend it and the rest of the fixings (omit the toppings) and stir.
2. Cover and place in the fridge overnight or at least four to six hours.
3. When ready to eat, garnish with the desired toppings and enjoy either warmed or at room temperature.

Chapter 4 - Lunches

There are so many options for lunch – from salads to soup; you are sure to find at least one week's worth of delicious ideas!

Arugula & Lentils Salad for One

Method of Storage: Refrigerator

This is what you'll need:

- ½ c. cooked - each:
-     -Quinoa
-     -Lentils
- 2 c. arugula
- ¾ c. roasted beets
- 2-4 tbsp. salad dressing

Instructions
1. Put the salad together, or as many as you want to prep.
2. Place in the fridge until ready to eat.

Asian Chopped Salad

Servings: 4
Method of Storage: Refrigerator

This is what you'll need:

- 1 medium of each bell pepper: Yellow and red
- 1 ½ c. shelled edamame
- 1 c. of each:
    -Shredded carrots
    -Thinly sliced snow peas
- 4 chopped scallions
- 4 c. of each:
    -Chopped romaine lettuce – 1 small head
    -Shredded purple cabbage – ½ small head

Instructions
1. Prepare the salads in four mason jars.
2. You can place 2 tablespoons of dressing into the bottom of each jar or pour it into individual containers.
3. Next, add the edamame, carrots, peppers, snow peas, scallions, lettuce, and cabbage.
4. Close the lid and refrigerate. When ready to eat, either shake the jar or plate the salad and add the dressing. How easy!

Avocado Chicken Wrap

Servings: 4-6 - varies
Method of Storage: Refrigerator

This is what you'll need:

- 2 cut & cubed avocados
- 4 c. chicken – cubed/shredded
- 1 t. garlic powder
- ½ t of each: salt and pepper
- 2 t. lime juice
- ¼ c. plain Greek yogurt
- ½ c. light mayonnaise
- Whole wheat tortillas

Instructions
1. Cut and cube the avocado and toss in a bowl with the prepared chicken.
2. Combine the seasonings, yogurt, and mayonnaise.
3. Cover with plastic wrap and refrigerate for a minimum of 30 minutes.
4. When ready to eat, spoon into the tortilla and fold over like a burrito.

Black Bean & Sweet Potato Salad

Servings: 2
Method of Storage: Refrigerator

This is what you'll need:

- 6 tbsp. Avocado dressing
- 2/3 c. roasted sweet potato cubes
- ½ c. seasoned black beans
- ½ c. purple cabbage
- 2/3 c. cooked quinoa
- 4 c. mixed salad greens

Instructions
1. Wash, dry, and cube the potato. Rub with some oil, salt, pepper, and garlic powder. Prepare the sweet potatoes in a 425ºF oven for 20-30 minutes. Let them cool.
2. Layer all of the fixings into two mason jars. Start with the dressing, cabbage, black beans, quinoa, sweet potato cubes, and mixed salad greens.
3. Store in the fridge and warm the chosen layers on a plate when it is time to serve – if you wish.

Butternut Chickpea Fajitas

Servings: 4
Method of Storage: Freezer up to 1 month

This is what you'll need:

- 1 can (19 oz.) chickpeas
- 4 c. butternut squash
- 1 sliced red onion
- 2 bell peppers
- ½ t. salt
- 1 tbsp. sugar
- 1 ½ t. of each:
    -Paprika
    -Cumin
- ½ t. garlic powder
- 2 tbsp. olive oil
- Juice of 1 lime

This is what you'll need for serving:

- Greek yogurt
- 8-12 (6-inch) tortillas
- Avocado
- Salsa
- Cilantro

Instructions
1. Drain and rinse the chickpeas. Cut the onions and squash into ½-inch strips.
2. Combine all of the fixings and place in a heavy-duty freezer bag.
   Shake well and freeze.

3. To Bake: Prepare the oven in advance to 425°F. Thaw the package of fajitas or the amount you want to eat. Bake 25 minutes – flipping about halfway through the baking process.
4. Enjoy whether you are on the run or at home relaxing!

Cauliflower Cashew Lunch Bowl

Servings: 4-6
Method of Storage: Refrigerator

This is what you'll need:

- 2/3 c. uncooked pearl barley (2 c. cooked)
- 8-10 cups - 1 head cauliflower – bite-sized pieces
- 1 tbsp. olive oil
- ¼ c. finely diced red onion
- ½ c. cashews
- 1 can chickpeas – rinsed & drained
- Pepper and salt to taste

Instructions
1. Prepare the barley according to the package directions.
2. Set the oven temperature ahead of time to 400°F.
3. Break the cauliflower apart and toss with the oil and a sprinkle of pepper and salt. Spread it out on a baking tin. Roast 30-45 minutes until browned and softened.
4. Add the cashews in another pan for about five minutes until golden. Cool the fixings.
5. Toss the salads together and add to five sealable lunch containers.
6. Store in the fridge until ready to use.

Chicken Fajita Lunch Bowls

Servings: 4
Method of Storage: Refrigerator

This is what you'll need for the chicken:

- 1 tbsp. olive oil
- 2 breasts of chicken
- Pepper & Salt

This is what you'll need for the salad:

- 2 bell peppers - strips
- ¾ c. uncooked basmati rice
- 1 c. corn kernels
- 2 tbsp. diced red onions

This is what you'll need for the vinaigrette:

- ½ t. of each:
- -Ground cumin
- -Paprika
- 1 t. chili powder
- 1 tbsp. of each:
- -Sugar
- -Lime juice
- ¼ t. salt
- 3 tbsp. of each:
- -Olive oil
- -White wine vinegar

Instructions

1. Warm up the oven to 425°F.
2. Arrange the chicken in a baking dish and give it a drizzle of oil. Sprinkle with the salt and pepper.
3. Bake ten minutes, flip and bake another 10-15 minutes until done. Let it rest ten minutes before slicing.

Prepare the lunch bowls:
1. Prepare and let the rice cool a few minutes. Combine with the peppers, onions, and corn.
2. Mix and shake the vinaigrette and add to the bowl – tossing well.
3. Divide into 4 lunch containers and add the chicken on top.
4. Place in the fridge until needed.

Chicken Salad

Servings: 2-3
Method of Storage: Refrigerator

This is what you'll need:

- 1 ½ c. diced chicken
- 12 green/red seedless grapes
- 3 tbsp. mayonnaise/more as needed to moisten
- ½ c. chopped celery
- 1 green chopped onion
- Pepper & Salt to taste

Instructions

1. Combine the celery, diced chicken, and green onion with the mayonnaise. Sprinkle with the pepper and salt – adding more mayo if needed
2. Chop the grapes into halves and mix in to combine. If desired, add a dash of curry powder.
3. You can use it as a filling for buns, rolls, or sliced bread, rolls. Make it even healthier and add it to heaps of lettuce leaves or greens. You can even add this to one of your mason jar salads.

Chickpea & Quinoa Salad

Servings: 2
Method of Storage: Refrigerator in a jar

This is what you'll need for the dressing:

- 2 tbsp. olive oil
- 1 t. of each:
- -Dijon mustard
- -Maple syrup
- Pepper & Salt – to taste
- ½ t. garlic powder
- Juice of 1 lemon

This is what you'll need for the salad:

- 1 c. of each:
- -Chickpeas – canned
- -Chopped cucumbers
- -Chopped cherry tomatoes
- -Cooked quinoa
- ½ c. chopped flat leaf parsley
- 3-4 c. arugula
- Also Needed: 2 wide-mouthed mason jars

Instructions
1. Prepare the dressing. Whisk all of the fixings together to your liking. Pour the dressing into a mason jar or two individual containers.
2. Divide the ingredients between the two jars in the order provided.
3. Close the lid and store in the fridge until ready to eat.
4. When ready to eat, just dump into a dish and enjoy!

Enchilada Lunch Bowls

Servings: 6-8
Method of Storage: Refrigerator

This is what you'll need:

- 1 small zucchini
- ½ small onion
- 1 red pepper
- 1 small summer squash
- 1 c. corn kernels
- 1 can of each:
- -19 oz. enchilada sauce
- -15 oz. black beans
- 1 c. shredded non-dairy cheese
- 6 corn tortillas
- 1 t. of each:
- -Olive oil
- -Paprika
- -Ground cumin
- -Garlic powder
- ¼ t. black pepper
- ¾ t. salt

- Also Needed: 4 (3-4 c.) Pyrex dishes/8-inch baking dish cut into 4th's

Instructions
1. Rinse and drain the beans, and dice the veggies. Chop the tortillas.
2. Set the oven temperature to warm up to 375°F.
3. Using the medium heat setting, pour the oil into a skillet and toss in the veggies. Saute five to seven minutes. Add

the beans and simmer another two minutes. Cool the
fixings and assemble the bowls.

4. Prepare the Bowl: 2 tbsp. sauce, ½ c. veggies, ¼ c. chopped
    corn tortillas, 1-2 tbsp. cheese, and 2 tbsp. sauce. Continue
    one more layer with cheese on the top (in each dish).

5. Arrange the bowls on a baking tin and bake about 20
    minutes until the cheese has melted. Remove and cool.
    Cover with a tight-fitting lid and refrigerate.

6. To Reheat: Bake 20 minutes at 375°F, or two minutes in the
    microwave.

Grilled Chicken Veggie Bowls

Servings: 8
Method of Storage: Refrigerator

This is what you'll need:
- 1 pkg. (16 oz. ea.) cooked:
- -Brown rice
- -Quinoa
- 4 c. (32 oz. ea.) roasted
- -Cauliflower florets
- -Chopped asparagus
- -Broccoli florets
- -Prepared Grilled Taco Lime Chicken – cubed – (see below for recipe)

Optional Alternatives – 4 c. each:
- -Roasted Brussels sprouts
- -Charred corn
- -Haricot verts

Instructions
1. Arrange ¼ cup each of the quinoa and brown rice into each container. Top off with 1 ½ c. of the cooked veggies. Be creative. Interchange the type of vegetables used in each of the bowls.
2. Add ½ c. of chicken to each one. Also, add some hot sauce or salsa – to your liking – after you reheat the bowl in the microwave.
3. Store in the fridge until you're ready to eat. Just microwave until heated and enjoy.
4. Tip: For roasting, place the veggies on a large baking dish and drizzle with a bit of oil. Give it a shake of pepper and salt.

5. Bake until fork tender at 375ºF. (The time varies depending on the veggies.)

Grilled Taco & Lime Chicken

Servings: 6-8
Method of Storage: Refrigerator/Freezer

This is what you'll need:

- 2 split limes
- 3-4 med.-large chicken breasts – no skin or bones
- 1 t. of each:
- -Kosher salt
- -Ground cumin
- ½ t. of each:
- -Garlic salt
- -Smoked/regular paprika
- -Freshly cracked black pepper

Instructions
1. Prepare the outdoor/indoor grill (med.-high).
2. Combine the garlic salt, pepper, salt, cumin, and paprika in a mixing container.
3. Use a large bowl/Ziploc-type bag and toss in the chicken and seasonings. Squeeze the lime juice from one of the lemons over the top. Mix and marinate for one to five hours. You can also grill at this time.
4. Lightly spray the grill when ready to cook. When done add to a large platter for ten minutes before slicing. When sliced, add the last of the lime over the top and enjoy as you like.
5. You can store in the fridge or freeze in portion containers for later use in your meal prepping plan.

Mango & Avocado Sushi Rolls

Servings: 5
Method of Storage: Refrigerator

This is what you'll need:

- 1 head riced cauliflower
- 1 piece of each:
    -Avocado
    -Cucumber
    -Purple cabbage
    -Mango
    -Carrots
- 5 Nori wrappers

Instructions
1. Thinly slice the fixings and rice the cauliflower.
2. Lay out the nori wrappers on the counter and add a layer of the rice to cover approximately 2/3 of the nori.
3. Add the veggies about ¾ of the way down the sheet.
4. Roll the wrapper tightly and dab with some water to seal the edge of the roll. Place on a serving dish and slice into rounds.
5. Put the covered container in the fridge until ready for lunch.

Mason Jar Salads

Jar salads are done in layers. This makes it easy to see your portions, what they contain and they are lovely to look at – you can write on the lid, the day you made the salad. You can get mason jars at any craft store, on Amazon or you save the jars from pickles and applesauce.

What is provided below is not set in stone; use the salad toppings that you like best and mix them any way you choose. These salads are a great go-to for meals in a hurry and are super portable for taking to work.

This is what you'll need:

- Large mason jar with lid
- Your favorite dressing
- Tomatoes, cucumbers, red onion, asparagus, celery, peppers, carrots, etc.
- Mushrooms, zucchini, beans, lentils, peas, corn, broccoli
- Boiled eggs and cheese (feta, gouda, cheddar, etc.)
- Rice, pasta, quinoa or couscous
- Nuts and greens as lettuce, spinach or arugula.

Instructions
1. Get all the ingredients ready; everything that needs to be cut, peeled, washed such as the veggies and fruits. Boil the pasta, quinoa or rice.
2. Once everything is laid out - chuck all the ingredients according to the layers (in the order listed) into the jars. As easy as that.

Southwestern Sweet Potato Lentil Jar Salad

Servings: 6
Method of Storage: Mason jars in the refrigerator – 4 days

This is what you'll need:

- 6 cups potato cubes
- ½ t. chili powder
- 1 tbsp. olive oil
- 1 can of each:
    -19 oz. brown lentils
    -11.5 oz. corn kernels
- 1 red bell pepper
- Dressing: Vinaigrette

Instructions
1. Prepare the oven to 425°F.
2. Toss the cubed sweet potatoes into the oil and chili powder.
3. Roast for 10 minutes, flip, and bake 15 minutes on the other side.
4. Prepare the jars:
    a. 1 tbsp. vinaigrette
    b. ½ c. lentils
    c. ½ c. corn
    d. 1 c. potato cubes
    e. Bell pepper slices
5. Close the lid and store in the fridge up to four days.

Sushi Jar – Deconstructed

Servings: 1
Method of Storage: Refrigerator

This is what you'll need:

- ¾ c. short grain brown rice
- 1 tbsp. seasoned sushi vinegar
- 4 sheets seasoned seaweed
- ¼ c. of each:
    -Cucumber matchsticks
    -Shredded carrot
- ½ diced avocado
- *Added Ingredients*
    -Pickled ginger
    -Lime juice

Instructions
1. Prepare the rice and place into a container. Pour the vinegar into the dish while it's warm. Let it cool.
2. Slice the seaweed into small strips or use a full sheet of nori.
3. Slice the cucumbers and carrots into matchsticks. Dice the avocado and lightly toss with the lime juice (preventing browning).
4. Layer each ingredient into the jar, any way you like. You can layer with the seaweed on the bottom and top with rice in between. Make your own pattern and enjoy!
5. Store in the fridge.

Turkey Taco Lunch Bowls

Now you can use some of the ingredients from the breakfast burritos. Layer all your favorite toppings into your containers and place in the fridge.

This is what you'll need:

- ¾ c. cooked rice
- Zest of 1 lime
- Pinch of salt
- 1 lb. ground turkey
- Chopped cilantro
- 1 pkg. taco seasoning of choice
- 1 can roasted corn
- Salsa of your choice
- Shredded cheese

Instructions:
1. Add the lime zest, salt and chopped cilantro to rice.
2. Cook turkey and taco seasoning, per package directions.
3. Assemble Taco bowls in your Tupperware (layer taco meat, roasted corn,
   salsa and shredded cheese; pop in the fridge until needed.

Soups

Apple Butternut Squash Soup

Yields: 3 quarts
Method of Storage: Frozen or Canned

This is what you'll need:

- 1 med./large butternut squash
- 1 tbsp. molasses - for the roasting of squash
- 2 large/3 small apples
- 2 small/med. onions
- 3 garlic cloves
- 2 qt. chicken broth – homemade
- 1/8 – ¼ t. cayenne pepper – optional
- Pepper & Sea salt – to taste

Instructions
1. Coarsely chop the onions, apples, and garlic.
2. Peel, deseed, and cube the squash. Scatter it over the baking sheet and toss with the melted butter, molasses, sea salt, and pepper. Roast for 40 minutes at 425°F.
3. Saute the apples and onion (med. temperature) in ¼ cup of butter along with a pinch of salt. Toss in the garlic for another minute, and add the broth roasted squash, and seasoning. Bring to a boil.
4. Lower the temperature to med-low, and slowly cook about five additional minutes. Puree thoroughly using a regular or immersion blender. Season to taste.
5. You can freeze or can the contents to keep your prep stock up to date.

Broccoli Soup

Servings: 7-8 quarts
Method of Storage: ½ gallon containers in the freezer or quart jars

This is what you'll need:

- 4 large carrots
- 4 lb. organic broccoli – 4 bunches/4 lb. bag frozen
- 4 small sliced onions
- 7 garlic cloves
- 1/3 c. fat – butter/lard/coconut oil
- ½ c. brown rice flour – optional for thickening or use a potato
- Sea salt and pepper – to taste
- 4 qt. chicken stock- homemade best

Instructions

1. Coarsely chop the veggies, including the broccoli stalks. Saute the carrots, broccoli, and onions along with a pinch of salt in the chosen fat for 10-15 minutes.
2. Toss in the garlic with the flour and saute one to two minutes. Pour in the stock. Once it boils, lower the heat and puree the soup using a blender.
3. Add a splash of coconut milk when serving.
4. Freeze what you don't have for your meal in quart or ½ gallon-sized containers, whichever one suits your needs the best.

Fresh Tomato Soup

Yields: 2 Quarts
Method of Storage: Refrigerator or freezer in ½ gallon containers

This is what you'll need:

- ¼ c. butter/lard/coconut oil – for cooking
- 2 large carrots
- 2 med. onions
- 3-4 garlic cloves
- 1 qt. chicken bone broth
- 2 tbsp. of each:
    -Basil
    -Organic tomato paste
- 5 large/6-7 small tomatoes/32 oz. can in winter months
- 2 t. molasses
- To Taste: Sea salt and pepper

Instructions
1. Saute the carrots and onions in a stock pot using the fat of choice. Add a pinch of salt, garlic, and tomato paste. Saute for one minute.
2. Blend in the tomatoes, stock, and basil. Bring to boil and reduce the heat. Continue cooking slowly for 25 minutes.
3. Remove from the heat and add the molasses.
4. Puree and serve or freeze in a ½ gallon or another container of your choice. Be sure to label the container.

Sweet Potato Peanut Stew

Servings: 6
Method of Storage: Refrigerator for 5 days – Freezer for 3 months

This is what you'll need:

- 1 c./3 ribs of celery
- 1 small onion
- 1 each bell peppers: red and green
- 3 garlic cloves
- 1 t. of each:
  -Ginger
  -Coriander
  -Cumin
  -Turmeric
- ¼ t. cinnamon
- 2 c. vegetable broth
- 1 can/homemade 28 oz. no-salt diced tomatoes – with the juices
- 3 c. sweet potatoes
- 1 can (19 oz.) chickpeas
- ¼ c. of each:
  -Pitted dates/raisins
  -Natural peanut butter
- ½ c. finely chopped cilantro
- 1 tbsp. lemon juice - freshly squeezed
- To Taste: White pepper and salt

Instructions

1. Prepare the Veggies: Peel the potato. Dice the celery and potatoes. Deseed the peppers and remove the pit from the dates or use raisins. Rinse and drain the chickpeas.

2. Stir in the celery, onion, and garlic along with ¼ cup of the vegetable broth in a large soup pot. Simmer about five minutes.

3. Stir in the spices and continue cooking for about another minute. Toss in the potatoes and peppers, stirring well.

4. Add the rest of the broth and tomatoes. Simmer uncovered about 20 minutes. Stir in the raisins/dates, chickpeas, lemon, peanut butter, and cilantro. Stir until well combined. Turn off the heat and let it cool.

5. You can serve now or store in the refrigerator for up to five days. You can also freeze this tasty soup for three months. What a tasty treat!

Chapter 5 - Dinners

Apricot Ginger Chicken

Servings: 4-5
Method of Storage: Freezer up to 3 months

This is what you'll need:

- 2/3 c. apricot jam
- 1 tbsp. low-sodium soy sauce
- 1 lb. thighs/breasts
- 1-inch ginger root – peeled & grated
- 3 minced garlic cloves
- 1 lb. frozen green beans

Instructions
1. Remove all of the bones and skin from the chicken and add into the bag. Then add the beans along with all of the fixings.
2. Squeeze out all of the air and seal. Lay flat in the freezer.
3. To Prepare: When ready, thaw in the fridge overnight/in a bowl of cold water. Add to a slow cooker and prepare on low for six hours until done.
4. Serve anytime!

Broccoli Quinoa Bowl for Dinner

Servings: 4-6
Method of Storage: Refrigerator

This is what you'll need

- 3 heads of broccoli – florets
- 6 c. cooked quinoa – 3 c. dried - approximately
- 3-4 peeled garlic cloves
- 1 lemon
- 1 c. blanched almonds
- 3 t. nutritional yeast
- Freshly cracked black pepper – to taste
- 1 t. salt

This is what you'll need for the topping:

- Sliced avocado
- ½ c. toasted slivered almonds
- Optional: Crushed red pepper flakes

Instructions
1. Prepare a large pot on the stove and chop the broccoli into bite-sized pieces. Cut the stem into 1-inch bits. Keep them separated.
2. Add the stems and cloves to the water and cook five to six minutes.
3. When tender, remove the cloves and stems from the water. Bag them.
4. Add the florets to the water and cook two minutes. Cool and bag them.
5. Soak the almonds at least one hour. Add ½ of the avocado, the soaked almonds (drain the water), salt, nutritional yeast, and 2 cups of water to a blender. Puree until smooth –

adding water ¼ cup at a time. Add pepper and salt to taste. Bag it.

6. When ready to prepare; toss in the pre-cooked quinoa and add with the broccoli mixture – cooking to warm it thoroughly. Drain through a fine-meshed strainer and return to the pot.

7. Set the containers of quinoa and broccoli mixes in the fridge until ready to eat.

8. Prepare the meal. Toast some almonds and slice the avocado. Combine and warm up the fixings. Add the desired toppings when served.

Chickpea & Butternut Fajitas

Servings: 4-6
Method of Storage: Freezer up to 1 month

This is what you'll need:

- 1 can (19 oz.) chickpeas
- 4 c. butternut squash
- 1 sliced red onion
- 2 bell peppers
- ½ t. salt
- 1 tbsp. of each
-     -Sugar
-     -Chili powder
- 1 ½ t. of each:
-     -Paprika
-     -Cumin
- ½ t. garlic powder
- Juice of 1 lime
- 2 tbsp. olive oil

This is what you'll need for serving:

- Greek yogurt
- 8-12 (6-inch) tortillas
- Avocado
- Salsa
- Cilantro

Instructions
1. Drain and rinse the chickpeas. Cut the onions and squash into ½-inch strips.

2. Combine all of the fixings and place in a heavy-duty
    freezer bag.
    Shake well and freeze.
3. To Bake: Prepare the oven in advance to 425°F. Thaw the
    package of fajitas or the amount you want to eat. Bake 25
    minutes – flipping about halfway through the baking
    process.
4. Enjoy whether you are on the run or at home relaxing!

Curried Chickpea Bowls

Servings: 3
Method of Storage: Refrigerator in glass dishes

This is what you'll need for the garlicky spinach:

- 1 t. avocado oil
- 3 minced garlic cloves
- ¼ t. sea salt
- 5 oz. baby spinach
- ½ lemon – juiced

This is what you'll need for the chickpeas:

- 2 minced garlic cloves
- 2 t. avocado oil
- 1 large chopped onion
- 1 can (15 oz.) chickpeas – rinsed & drained
- 1 t. cumin
- 2 t. curry
- ½ t. cinnamon
- 2 tbsp. tomato paste
- 3 tbsp. water
- ½ t. of each – Pepper & Sea salt

This is what you'll need for the topping:

- Chopped green onion
- Chopped fresh cilantro
- 3 c. cooked brown rice

Also needed: 3 glass storage containers

Instructions

1. Prepare the rice and warm up one teaspoon of oil in a skillet using the medium heat setting. Toss in the garlic and saute one or two minutes. Add the spinach and continue sautéing for another 2-3 minutes or until it wilts. Sprinkle with the salt and lemon juice. Toss and remove from the heat and add to a small dish.
2. Add the onions and garlic along with another of the oil to the skillet and simmer another five minutes. Sprinkle in the spices, tomato paste, and chickpeas. Toss and add the water. Sprinkle with the pepper and salt, tossing another two to three minutes. Remove from the heat.
3. Allow the fixings to cool.
4. Prepare the containers with 1 cup of rice and 1/3 each of the chickpeas and baby spinach. Top each one off with the green onion and cilantro. Cover and place in the refrigerator until time to use.

Greek Chicken

Servings: 4
Method of Storage: Refrigerator for Lunches

This is what you'll need:

- 1 c. Greek yogurt – whole milk
- 1 cucumber
- 2 ½ t. salt – divided
- 1 t. garlic powder – divided
- 3 tbsp. extra-virgin olive oil – divided
- 1 tbsp. of each:
-   -White vinegar
-   -Dill – see note
- 1 lb. chicken breasts 4 (4 oz.) skinless and boneless
- ¾ tbsp. Italian seasoning
- ½ t. of cach:
-   -Paprika
-   -Cornstarch
-   -Onion powder
-   -Black pepper
- ¼ t. ground of each:
-   -Nutmeg
-   -Cinnamon
- 1 c. dried farro/brown rice
- 15-20 of each:
-   -Quartered cherry tomatoes
-   -Chopped – pitted – halved black olives
- ¼ diced red onion
- 1 juiced lemon
- 1 tbsp. red wine vinegar
- Non-stick cooking spray

Note: You can use dill paste, dried dill weed, or freshly minced dill paste.

Instructions
1. Prepare the Tzatziki: Grate ½ of the cucumber and place it in a mesh strainer. Squeeze out the excess water using paper towels and add to a medium mixing bowl. Toss with the yogurt, 2 tbsp. of the oil, ½ teaspoon of salt and garlic powder along with 1 tablespoon each of the dill and vinegar. Stir and chill in the fridge.
2. Set the oven to 450°F. Use parchment paper or aluminum foil to line a baking sheet. Also, spray it with the oil spray.
3. Make the Seasoning: Combine the following:
    a. ¾ tbsp. of the Italian seasoning, 1 t. salt and 1 t. garlic powder.
    b. Also add ½ t. of each: pepper, paprika, cornstarch, onion powder, and pepper. Add ¼ t. nutmeg and cinnamon.
4. Arrange the chicken portions on the baking tin and coat with the Greek seasoning. Spray again with the cooking oil. Bake 15-20 minutes or until done.
5. Prepare the farro and make the Greek salad. Dice the second half of the cucumber, quarter the tomatoes, chop the olives, and dice the onion. Combine all of the fixings in a large container.
6. Sprinkle with the salt and pepper, oil, vinegar, and juice of a lemon. Stir.
7. Portion the fixings into four containers with 1 breast, ½ cup of farro, ¼ of the salad, and ¼ of the tzatziki.
8. Cover and store in the fridge for lunch all week long!

Power Bowl Essentials

Servings: 1 meal
Method of Storage: Refrigerator

This is what you'll need:

- 2 c. greens
- 1 medium orange yam sweet potato
- ½ c. black beans
- 1 tbsp. chosen dressing
- Pepper & salt to taste

Instructions
1. Wash the kale and greens. Remove the stems from the greens. Drain and rinse the beans.
2. Set the oven temperature to 400°F.
3. Poke several holes in the potato and microwave about two minutes. Slice into bite-sized bits. Roast 20 minutes until the edges are crispy.
4. Steam the greens about 5 minutes in a splash of water until bright green.
5. Cool the ingredients and place each of the fixings into a serving dish.
6. Cover and refrigerate until ready to eat.
7. Serve with a tasty dressing.

Quinoa Green Burritos

Servings: 6
Method of Storage: Refrigerator or freezer

This is what you'll need:

- 1 avocado
- 2 garlic cloves
- 4 trimmed scallions
- Handful – basil/chives/cilantro – or all
- ¼ c. of each:
- -Almond butter/tahini
- -Water
- 5 tbsp. lemon juice
- Coconut Aminos/salt – to taste
- Optional: 1 serrano chili pepper

- Kale – 2 bunches
- 6 multi-grain/spinach tortillas
- 3 c. of each:
- -Cooked mung beans
- -Cooked quinoa
- Optional: Hemp seeds or toasted pepitas

Instructions
1. Use a food processor/blender and combine the garlic, avocado, herbs, scallion, tahini, lemon juice, water, serrano, and salt. Pulse until smooth and add to a mason jar.
2. Add the kale in a large container with about ½ of the dressing. Coat well.
3. Fill one tortilla with about ½ cup each of the mung beans, quinoa, and a dollop of the dressing. Toss in a handful of the hemp seeds/pepitas. Simply fold and roll.

4. For storage, just wrap them in parchment paper and foil.
    Place in the fridge or freeze in multiples using a large
    plastic freezer bag.

Ramen Noodle Salad

Servings: 5
Method of Storage: Refrigerator

This is what you'll need:

- 1 pkg. (8 oz.) organic rice ramen noodles
- 1 c grated carrots
- 3 c. shredded red cabbage
- 5 sliced scallion stalks
- ¼ c. slivered almonds

This is what you'll need for the special sauce:

- ½ lime – juiced
- 3 tbsp. of each:
- -Warm water
- -Apple cider vinegar
- 2 tbsp. of each
- -Tamari
- -Maple syrup
- ½ t. of each:
- -Onion powder
- -Garlic powder
- ¼ c. smooth – room temperature- peanut butter

Instructions
1. Prepare the salads into individual dishes or leave it in the serving dish.
2. Whisk the dressing ingredients together and add water to get the right consistency (just a little at a time).
3. If you know you will be in a hurry, also add the dressing into individual containers.

4. Note: Prepare the noodles the day before using and add a small amount of olive oil before placing them in the refrigerator.
5. This is a very flexible preparation item. Enjoy!

Roasted Sausage with Vegetables

This is what you'll need:

- 1 lb. fingerling potatoes
- ¾ lb. green beans or asparagus
- 4 links bratwurst or mild Italian sausage
- 4 tbsp. olive oil
- 4 carrots (peeled)
- 1 small pkg. cherry tomatoes
- 1 bell pepper (yellow or red) sliced
- Salt & Pepper to taste

Instructions

1. Line the pan with foil.
2. Cut bratwurst/sausage into quarters.
3. Place all vegetables and meat onto a sheet pan. Cover with olive oil, salt, and pepper. Mix with your hands until everything is coated.
4. Bake in the oven at 350°F for 35 min, or until potatoes are tender and meat is cooked thoroughly.

This is a great go-to you can spread out over several containers and mix and match with those Mason Jar Salads.

Southwestern Black Bean Couscous Salad

Servings: 4-6
Method of Storage: Refrigerator

This is what you'll need:

- 1 ¼ c. Israeli couscous
- 1 ½ c. water
- 1 can (15 oz.) rinsed black beans
- 1 c. of each:
- -Quartered cherry tomatoes
- -Sweet corn
- ½ red finely diced onion

Instructions
1. Pour the water into a pot. When it starts boiling, add the couscous and lower the heat. Simmer until the water is absorbed. Add to a plastic closed container and chill.
2. Add the black beans, couscous, corn, onion, and tomato in separate containers and place in the fridge.
3. They are ready when you are, just add the desired dressing!

Tahini Harissa Buddha Bowl

Servings: 1
Method of Storage: Refrigerator

This is what you'll need:

- ½ c. of each:
- -Cooked lentils
- -Cooked quinoa
- 1 c. raw arugula
- ¾ c. roasted sweet potatoes
- 1 tbsp. of each:
- -Tahini
- -Spicy harissa

Instructions
1. Arrange the desired amount of bowls on the counter and fill with the arugula, potatoes, lentils, and quinoa.
2. Cover and place in the fridge.
3. When it's time to eat, top off with the harissa, and a drizzle of the tahini.

Tofu Burrito Bowl

Servings: 5
Method of Storage: Refrigerator – 10 days

This is what you'll need:

- 1 pkg. (14 oz.) extra-firm tofu
- 2 tbsp. olive oil
- ½ t. of each:
    -Cayenne
    -Paprika
    -Garlic powder
    -Chili powder
    -Pepper
    -Sea salt
    -Chipotle powder

This is what you'll need for the toppings:

- Avocado
- Greens – kale/spinach/romaine
- Black beans
- Tomatoes/salsa
- Red onion
- Cilantro

Instructions
1. Drain the tofu between paper towels to remove the liquid.
2. Prepare a large skillet over medium heat. Add the tofu and chop it apart. Add the seasonings and cook 8-10 minutes.
3. Cool and portion the tofu into the meal prep container of choice. Arrange the chosen toppings to the side.
4. Store in the fridge for up to ten days.

5. You can also add a batch of quinoa to go along with this delicious bowl.

Soup

Chicken Soup in the Pot

Servings: 6
Method of Storage: Refrigerator

This is what you'll need:

- 6 chicken thighs (bone and skin on)
- 1 bag baby-size of each:
  -Carrots
  -Spinach
- 3 stalks chopped celery
- 1 yellow - chopped onion
- 1 container mushrooms
- 4 tbsp. olive oil
- To Taste: Pepper and salt
- 4 leaves finely chopped fresh sage
- 2 tbsp. finely chopped fresh rosemary
- 2 t. thyme
- 10 minced cloves garlic
- 1 box low sodium chicken broth or stock
- Water as needed

Instructions
1. In a large crockpot add all ingredients, except the spinach. Pour chicken stock into the crockpot, until chicken is covered if there is not enough stock to cover chicken completely, add a little water.
2. Turn crockpot on high and let cook all day, you can set it and forget it.
3. Soup is done when chicken falls off the bones with a light prodding with a fork.

4. Separate all the bones (dispose of) from the meat and stir it
    a little to break up the meat into smaller pieces.
5. Add the spinach and stir until it's wilted down.

At this point, it's done as is, or you can add rice, noodles or
dumplings. This makes a great dinner or lunch; it's especially nice
for quick meals, you can heat up an individual minute rice cup and
drop in your bowl of soup to keep from having to put rice in the
whole pot. I've also found this is super good with a couple garlic
breadsticks; you can never go wrong with garlic and butter.

Freeze and save for later!

Creamy Vegetable Soup

Yields: 2 (+) gallons
Method of Storage: Refrigerator, canning jars or freezer

This is what you'll need:

- 5 chopped medium onions
- ¼ c. butter/coconut oil/tallow/lard – for cooking
- 8 minced garlic cloves
- 4 qt. chicken bone broth – homemade
- 5 lb. bag mixed veggies
- 8 med. chopped potatoes
- To Taste: Salt and pepper

Instructions
1. Coarsely chop the vegetables. Saute the onions in a stock pot with the butter about eight minutes. Add a few pinches of salt and add the garlic – cooking one minute.
2. Pour in the broth, potatoes, and veggies. Lower the heat and simmer five to ten minutes. Ladle out ½ of the soup in a container and puree either with an immersion or blender. Add it back to the pot and stir to combine.
3. Season to taste. Enjoy some now or prep it all in the freezer using plastic containers. Freeze without the lids for about 24 hours until completely frozen. Lastly, place the lids.

Mason Jar Pho Soup

Servings: 1
Method of Storage: Refrigerator

This is what you'll need:

- ½ c. of each:
-   -Julienned red pepper
-   -Thinly sliced carrot
- 1 t. freshly minced of each:
-   -Garlic
-   -Ginger
- ¼ c. chopped green onion
- 1 c. thin rice noodles – uncooked
- 1/8 c. soy sauce – gluten-free
- 3 c. chicken/vegetable stock
- Also Needed: 1 large mason jar

Instructions
1. Prepare the veggies and add to the mason jar – the carrots, peppers,
   garlic, ginger, green onion, and noodles – in that order.
2. Time to Eat: Pour in the boiling chicken stock and soy sauce.
3. Tighten the lid and let it sit for about 10 to 15 minutes. The veggies and noodles should be tender.

Peanut & Sweet Potato Stew

Servings: 6
Method of Storage: Refrigerator for 5 days/Freezer for 3 months

This is what you'll need:

- 1 c./3 ribs of celery
- 1 small onion
- 1 each bell peppers: red and green
- 3 garlic cloves
- 1 t. of each:
- -Ginger
- -Coriander
- -Cumin
- -Turmeric
- ¼ t. cinnamon
- 2 c. vegetable broth
- 1 can/homemade 28 oz. no-salt diced tomatoes – with the juices
- 3 c. sweet potatoes
- 1 can (19 oz.) chickpeas
- ¼ c. of each:
- -Pitted dates/raisins
- -Natural peanut butter
- ½ c. finely chopped cilantro
- 1 tbsp. lemon juice - freshly squeezed
- To Taste: White pepper and salt

Instructions
1. Prepare the Veggies: Peel the potato. Dice the celery and potatoes. Deseed the peppers and remove the pit from the dates or use raisins. Rinse and drain the chickpeas.

2. In a large soup pot (med. setting) toss in the celery, the onion, and garlic along with ¼ cup of the vegetable broth. Simmer about five minutes.
3. Stir in the spices and continue cooking for about another minute. Toss in the potatoes and peppers, stirring well.
4. Add the rest of the broth and tomatoes. Simmer uncovered about 20 minutes. Stir in the raisins/dates, chickpeas, lemon, peanut butter, and cilantro. Stir until well combined. Turn off the heat and let it cool.
5. You can serve now or store in the refrigerator for up to five days. You can also freeze for up to three months.

Tortilla & Chickpea Soup

Servings: 4-6
Method of Storage: Freezer

This is what you'll need:

- 1 c. salsa
- ¼ t. salt
- 1 t. of each:
- -Chili powder
- -Cumin
- 1 can of each drained:
- -Corn/fresh 15 oz.
- -Chickpeas – rinsed – 19 oz.
- 1 chopped onion
- 3 minced garlic cloves
- 4 c. vegetable stock

This is what you'll need for serving:

- 1 tbsp. lime juice
- Avocado
- Greek yogurt
- Tortilla chips
- Cilantro

Instructions
1. Prepare the soup and freeze. Use a large freezer bag to combine the cumin, salsa, salt, chili powder, chickpeas, onion, corn, and garlic. Remove the air from the bag and label with the date and contents. Freeze up to three months.
2. Time to Eat: Thaw for 24 hours in the refrigerator. Dump the bag into a five-quart slow cooker along with 4 cups of

stock. Prepare on the low setting for six to eight hours or high for three to four hours.
3. Stir in the lime juice right before serving along with the desired toppings.
4. This is perfect to drop into the pot on the way out of the door as you head off for a busy day!

Chapter 6 – Lunch Box Specials

You know how mornings can be when you just cannot get it together. Just grab one of these for lunch and go.

Avocado Chickpea Salad Collard Wraps

Servings: 2-3
Method of Storage: Refrigerator

This is what you'll need:

- 1 ½ c. chickpeas – (1) 15 oz. can
- 1 ripe avocado
- 1 med. celery stalk
- 1 med. carrot
- 1 large bell pepper
- ¼ c. cilantro
- 1 juiced lemon
- To Taste
- -½ t. salt
- -¼ t. pepper
- 6 collard green leaves

Instructions
1. Mash the avocado in a small dish.
2. Rinse and drain the chickpeas. Mash and combine them into a large mixing container with the celery, carrots, and bell pepper. Mix and add the lemon juice, mashed avocado, pepper, salt, and cilantro. Stir well.

3. Lay one of the leaves on the cutting board.
    Scoop out 1/3 to ½ cup of the chickpea salad
    on the leaf center. Make them all and store
    in the fridge.
4. They will last nicely up to five days in an
    air-tight container.

Ham & Cheese Croissant

Servings: 1
Method of Storage: 12 hrs. - Approx. in the fridge
together/freezer if longer

This is what you'll need:

- 2 thin slices (2 oz.) deli ham
- 1 plain croissant
- ½ small pear – 1/3 c. approx.
- 2 t. Dijon mustard
- ½ c. watercress – washed – dried – stems removed
- 2 thin slices (1 oz.) Muenster cheese

Instructions
1. Slice the croissant in half – horizontally.
2. Add all of the fixings to the sandwich and wrap in plastic wrap.
3. You can leave this in the fridge for about 12 hours/overnight. If you want it to be prepped ahead of time for more servings, just add the wet fixings in separate containers and prepare as needed. Enjoy either way!

Peanut Butter – Banana & Honey Sandwich

Servings: 1 Sandwich
Method of Storage: Refrigerator/freezer

This is what you'll need for the sandwich:

- 2 slices whole wheat bread
- 4 tbsp. organic creamy peanut butter
- 1 ripe banana
- 1 ½ tbsp. orange blossom honey

This is what you'll need for the carrot chips and dip:

- 4 large carrots
- 2 t. olive oil
- 1/3 c. Greek yogurt
- 2 t. sea salt
- 1 stem dill
- 1 cucumber

This is what you'll need for the chocolate covered apples:

- Chocolate dip mix
- 1 granny smith apple

Instructions
1. Core and slice the apple and dip them into chocolate. Arrange the slices on a paper plate covered with wax paper and place in the freezer to harden.
2. Prepare the oven in advance to 350°F.
3. Use a mandolin/thin slicer to slice the carrots paper-thin. Mix with the salt and

olive oil. Don't over-lap but place them on 2
baking sheets. Bake 30 minutes; rotating the
pan about halfway through the time (15 min.
or so).
4. When done, arrange on a platter to crisp.
5. Prepare the dip by finely chopping half of
   the cucumber and dicing the dill.
6. Combine the mixture with the salt and
   yogurt.
7. Make the sandwich with the fixings and
   enjoy every morsel!
8. Note: To make the process faster, you can
   use a microwavable chocolate mix or other
   substitutes. You can leave the fixings in the
   freezer/refrigerator until ready to prepare, so
   prep as many as you like.

Pesto Chicken Pita Pockets

Servings: 4
Method of Storage: Refrigerator

This is what you'll need for the chicken:

- 2 large breasts of chicken
- Pepper and salt to taste
- 1 tbsp. olive oil

This is what you'll need for the veggies:
6 cups in chunks:
- -Bell pepper
- -Red onion
- -Zucchini
- 1 tbsp. oil
- Pepper & salt

This will also be needed:

- 4 pita pockets
- 1/3 c. pesto

Instructions
1. Program the oven setting to 425°F.
2. Arrange the chicken in a baking pan along with the oil, salt, and pepper.
3. Toss in the veggies and more oil, pepper, and salt, in another pan.
4. Roast 10 minutes, flip, and continue cooking for another 10-15 minutes – to your liking.
5. For the chicken, give it another 15 minutes and let it rest ten minutes before slicing into strips.

6. Add the fixings in the pita, place in plastic,
    and refrigerate for later.
7. When ready to serve, slice in half, and
    enjoy!

Stuffed Bagel Sandwiches

Servings: 1-2
Method of Storage: Refrigerator

This is what you'll need:

- 2 small/2 large bagel
- ¼ c. whipped cream cheese
- 2 large slices – diced salami
- 2 tbsp. dill relish
- 4 diced baby carrots
- 1/8 t. of Salt and pepper
- Pinch of garlic powder to taste

Instructions
1. Slice the bagel down the middle and remove most of the inside breading to shape into a ring.
2. Combine the rest of the fixings in a container and mix well with a stand/hand mixer.
3. Fill the bagel with the mixture and place the second half on top.
4. Cut in half and serve.
5. For the prep; just don't put the sandwich together until ready to serve.

Chapter 7: Desserts

Now, comes the yummy menu items!

Almond Butter - Brown Rice Crispy Treats

Servings: 9
Method of Storage: Fridge or Freezer

This is what you'll need:

- 4 c. sprouted brown rice crisps
- ½ c. of each
-   -Almond butter
-   -Brown rice syrup
-   -Mini chocolate chips
- 1 t. vanilla extract
- Pinch of salt
- Also Needed: 9x9-inch cake pan

Instructions
1. Spray the pan with coconut oil cooking spray and place to the side.
2. In a large container – mix the brown syrup, almond butter, and salt until well combined. Stir in the rice crisps until coated; then add the mini chips. Stir well.
3. Arrange the concoction on the cake pan and press down using a spatula.
4. For the Prep: Place in the freezer for a minimum of 1 hour. Use a sharp knife to remove them and slice into nine squares.

Either store them in the refrigerator or sliced (9 pieces) and back into the freezer.

Chia Seed & Ginger Grapefruit Pudding

Servings: 2 Servings
Method of Storage: Refrigerator

This is what you'll need:

- ½ c. (from the can) full-fat coconut milk
- 6-7 chia seeds
- 1 ½ c. non-dairy unsweetened milk ex. cashew
- 1 t. of each:
-   -Vanilla extract
-   -Freshly grated ginger
- 1-3 t. pure maple syrup to taste

This is what you need for the topping:

- 2 large grapefruits – segmented
- ¼ c. toasted – unsweetened – flaked coconut

Instructions
1. Prepare the pudding. Shake or whisk all of the fixings in a jar/bowl.
2. Cover and place in the fridge for a minimum of two hours to thicken – shaking/mixing occasionally.
3. At that point, add seeds one tablespoon at a time (½ hr. in between).
4. Place in the fridge until ready to eat. Then, add the toppings when ready to eat.

Donuts in a Minute

This is what you'll need:

- 2 tubes biscuit dough (I really do think Pillsbury is the best here)
- ½ c. granulated sugar
- 1 tbsp. cinnamon
- 1 bottle vegetable oil
- Paper lunch bag

Instructions
1. In a large pot, heat the oil until it's in frying temperature. You can usually gauge this by flipping a very small drop of water at the oil. If it sizzles, you're ready to go. If not - let it heat longer.
2. Unroll the tubes of dough and separate into biscuit sections; using a small round cookie cutter about the size of a quarter (or a soda bottle top), press out the biscuit centers.
3. Fill the lunch bag with sugar and cinnamon, roll the top down to seal, and give the bag a good shake to incorporate cinnamon evenly.
4. Drop biscuit dough into hot oil and cook on both sides till golden brown and puffed up, use a slotted spoon to remove from oil.
5. Drop hot donuts into the bag and shake to coat.
6. You can, or jazz it up with a side of Nutella.

Gingerbread Granola

Yields: 5-6 Cups
Method of Storage: Countertop or Fridge

This is what you'll need:

- 1 ½ c. raw walnuts/pecans
- 4 c. old-fashioned rolled oats
- 1 t. fine-grain sea salt
- ½ t. of each:
-    -Ground ginger
-    -Cinnamon
- ½ c. olive oil/melted coconut oil
- ¼ c. molasses
- 1/3 c. real maple syrup
- ¾ t. vanilla
- ½ c. large coconut flakes – unsweetened
- 1/3 c. of each:
-    -Candied ginger
-    -Dried cranberries

Instructions
1. Set the oven temperature to 350ºF. Line a ½-sheet pan with a piece of parchment paper. Chop the cranberries and candied ginger.
2. Combine the nuts, oats, ginger, cinnamon, and salt, in a large bowl. Stir.
3. Blend in the syrup, oil, molasses, and vanilla. Dump the granola into the pan, and spread out in an even layer.
4. Bake 20 minutes, remove and add the coconut flakes. Blend in and return to the oven for ten more minutes.

5. After that time, remove the pan and add the
    ginger and cranberries. Stir again. Let it cool
    well.
6. Store on the shelf for one or two weeks;
    longer if in the fridge.

Parfaits on the Go

Servings: 6
Method of Storage: Plastic containers & plastic
bags in the refrigerator – 1 week

Ingredients
- 6 c. Greek yogurt
- 1 pint of each:
- -Blackberries
- -Raspberries
- -Blueberries
- 1 pkg. fresh pomegranate seeds
- 1 c. sliced almonds
- c. cornflakes/granola/favorite cereal

Also Needed: 6 plastic containers with lids

Instructions
1. Layer the contents starting with the yogurt, fruit, cereal, and lastly the almonds. Place in the fridge in an air-tight container. Cover each parfait tightly and enjoy during the week.
2. *Special Note*: All you need to do is portion the cereal and almonds in a separate baggie so they can remain fresh. Add to the jar before eating.

Peanut Butter & Chocolate Baked Oatmeal Cups

Servings: 12
Method of Storage: Refrigerator

This is what you'll need:

- 6 tbsp. water (+) 2 tbsp. chia seeds
- 3 med. to large bananas
- 1 c. unsweetened cashew/almond/coconut milk - ex. Silk
- ½ t. vanilla extract
- ¼ c. of each:
- -Creamy peanut butter
- -Pure maple syrup/15 drops liquid stevia
- 1 scoop chocolate plant-based protein powder –
  Example - Vega Chocolate Protein (+) Greens
- 2 tbsp. cocoa powder
- 3 c. old-fashioned oats
- Pinch of salt
- 1 tbsp. baking powder

Instructions
1. Set the oven temperature to 350ºF. Prepare the muffin tin with some cooking spray.
2. Toss the seeds in with the water to make the 'chia eggs.'
3. Smash the ripened bananas in a large container. Pour in the milk, stevia/syrup, peanut butter, and vanilla. Mix well and blend in the chia eggs to the mixture. Fold in the oats, protein powder, cocoa powder, salt, and baking powder. Stir well.

4. Spoon the batter into the tins. Bake 25
    minutes. Transfer the cups from the muffin
    tin and place on a cooling rack until
    completely cool.
5. Store in the fridge in an air-tight container.
    You can also freeze a few, (if they last that
    long)!
6. Enjoy for breakfast or as a quick snack full
    of nutritious fixings.

Peanut Butter Muffins

Servings: 12
Method of Storage: Air-tight container in the fridge
– 4 days

This is what you'll need:

- 1 c. natural peanut butter
- 2 med. bananas
- 6 Medjool dates – pits removed

Instructions
1. Set the oven temperature to 350°F. Grease or line a standard-sized muffin tin. Silicone liners are a great tool.
2. Combine the fixings in a food processor and blend well.
3. Spoon the batter into the muffin pans and bake 15-20 minutes.
4. Cool and store in the fridge. They are delicious for about four days.

Acai Bowls

Acai is a grape-like fruit which is native to South
America. This is simply a frozen
Acai pulp that is blended with berries and fruits. It
is topped off with all kinds of
goodies. The Acai unsweetened frozen packs are
available at some superstores
including Walmart.

To use each of the packets, simply run the acai pack
under the tap water (5 seconds or so) to break apart
the pulp into smaller pieces.

Green Tropical Bowl

Servings: 2
Method of Storage: Refrigerator

This is what you'll need:

- 2 c. fresh each:
-     -Kale
-     -Spinach
- 1 banana
- 7 oz. pkg. unsweetened acai berry pulp
- 1 c. of each:
-     -Frozen mango chunks
-     -Unsweetened almond milk

This is what you will need for the topping:

- 1 small sliced banana
- ½ c. granola – optional
- 4 tbsp. peeled & chopped pineapple
- 1-2 tbsp. shredded coconut - unsweetened
- Molasses

Instructions

1. Prepare the acai puree using a blender. Toss in the kale, spinach, acai pulp, banana, mango, and a bit of milk.
2. Blend slowly at first until chunks are reduced, and increase the speed until you reach high (another 15-20 seconds). Pour into two bowls and add the toppings. Garnish and cover until ready to eat.

Peanut Butter Loco Hawaiian

Servings: 2
Method of Storage: Refrigerator

This is what you'll need:

- 1 small banana
- 2 tbsp. cocoa powder
- 3 t. natural unsalted peanut butter
- 7 oz. acai pack berry pulp – unsweetened
- 1 c. of each:
- -Frozen strawberries
- -Unsweetened milk – almond

This is what you'll need for the toppings:

- 1 sliced small banana
- ½ c. granola – optional
- 2 tbsp. cocoa nibs
- 4 t. unsweetened coconut – shredded
- 3 t. natural unsalted peanut butter
- Drizzle of molasses - optional

Instructions
1. Using a blender combine the ingredients in the acai puree list (peanut butter, banana, cocoa powder, strawberries, acai pulp, and a splash of milk).
2. Divide the ingredients into 2 bowls. Place a cover on each one and place in the fridge until ready to serve or eat on the go.

Rainbow Bowl

Servings: 2
Method of Storage: Refrigerator

This is what you'll need for the puree:

- 1 small banana
- 7 oz. pkg. unsweetened acai berry pulp
- 1 c. frozen of each:
- -Blueberries
- -Strawberries
- 1 c. vanilla almond milk – unsweetened

This is what you'll need for the toppings:

- ½ c. blueberries
- 1 kiwi
- 1 small banana
- ½ c. of each:
- -Sliced strawberries
- -Mango/pineapple

- Optional: Granola – ½ c.
- Drizzle of molasses

Instructions
1. Peel the banana and pineapple. Chop the kiwi, pineapple, and banana into pieces.
2. Add the fixings (in the order given) to a blender. Begin on the slow setting until the chunks are broken apart. Increase the speed and add the milk in small increments.
3. When creamy, add the toppings.
4. Chill until ready to eat!

Ice Tray Smoothies

Each of the recipes in this category is specifically made by freezing the plain non-fat yogurt into ice cube trays. Once frozen, they are placed in freezer bags to accompany your favorite fruits. Then, simply prepare the chosen fruits and place them into Ziploc bags or containers; ready to go when you are! When ready to drink, just add the liquid, and you are in business!
Enjoy these anytime:

Coconut Water & Mixed Berry Smoothie

Servings: 1
Method of Storage: Freezer and fridge

This is what you'll need:

- ¼ c. frozen of each:
- -Mango chunks
- -Pineapple chunks
- -Strawberries
- -Blackberries
- 2 cubes frozen yogurt
- 1 c. coconut water

Instructions
1. Make as many as you want!

2. Prepare the fruit in a Ziploc type bag and place in the freezer. Be sure to mark the packages with a date and time clearly.
3. When ready to serve, just add the yogurt cubes, frozen fruit, and coconut water into a blender. Puree.
4. Serve with a smile!

Mango & Pineapple Yogurt Smoothie

Servings: 1
Method of Storage: Freezer and refrigerator

This is what you'll need:

- ½ c. frozen pineapple chunks
- ¾ c. frozen mango chunks
- 2 frozen cubes of yogurt
- 1 c. coconut water

Instructions
1. Prepare the fruit into chunks and add to baggies. Place in the baggies in the fridge (labeled).
2. When ready to drink; take the frozen cubes from the freezer, add the bag of fruit, and coconut water.
3. Puree in a blender and enjoy!

Chilly One-Serving Smoothies

The greatest part of preparing a smoothie in a freezer baggie is evident. You can make your own combinations. They are a great breakfast treat and a quick snack any time of the day or night!

Chocolate Chip Mint Smoothie

Method of Storage: Freezer

This is what you'll need:

- ½ diced avocado
- 1 med. banana
- 2 tbsp. of each:
- -Cacao powder
- -Cacao nibs
- ¼ c. fresh mint
- 1 c. spinach
- 1 ½ c. unsweetened chocolate almond milk – ex. Almond Breeze

Instructions
1. Combine the avocado, banana, mint, spinach, along with the cacao nibs and powder in a small freezer bag. Place it in the freezer until ready to use.
2. To Eat: Add the pack along with the milk, blending until smooth. Yummy!

Green Tropical Smoothie

Method of Storage: Freezer

This is what you'll need:

- 3 tbsp. hemp seeds
- 1 c. fresh each:
-    -Pineapple
-    -Mango
- 1 ½ c. unsweetened vanilla almond coconut blend – Almond Breeze

Instructions
1. Combine the fruit in a baggie and store it in the freezer.
2. When it's time to drink your treat, simply toss the fixings into the blender along with the milk, and blend until creamy smooth to your liking.

__Mixed Berry__

Method of Storage: Freezer

This is what you'll need:

- ½ c. fresh each of:
- -Raspberries
- -Blueberries
- 1 c. fresh strawberries
- 1 ½ c. unsweetened vanilla almond coconut blend – ex. Almond Breeze

Instructions
1. Combine all of the berries in a Ziploc baggie and place them in the freezer.
2. When ready to serve, pour in the almond milk with the berries, and blend until creamy smooth.

Strawberries & Chocolate

Servings: 1
Method of Storage: Freezer

This is what you'll need:

- 2 c. fresh strawberries
- 1 med. banana
- 1 ½ c. unsweetened chocolate almond milk
  – ex. Almond Breeze

Instructions
1. Toss all of the fruit fixings into a Ziploc
   type freezer bag.
2. Place the bag in the freezer until ready to
   blend. At that time, open the package, add it
   to the blender along with the milk, and mix
   until smooth.

Other Tasty Smoothies

Banana Strawberry & Green Smoothie

Servings: 4
Method of Storage: Freezer bags

This is what you'll need:

- 4 cups spinach
- 4 t. chia seeds
- 2 c. of each:
- -Whole strawberries
- -Sliced bananas

This is what you'll need for blending:
- 1 scoop - vanilla protein powder
- ½ - 1 c. almond milk - unsweetened

Instructions
1. Prepare a baking sheet with parchment paper.
2. Arrange the bananas and berries on the pan. Freeze until solid – about two hours.
3. Label four quart-sized freezer bags with the date and name of the smoothie.
4. Pour in one cup of fruit, one teaspoon of the seeds, and a handful of spinach to each bag. Seal and freeze.
5. When ready to use, add the milk and protein scoop. Enjoy!

Pina-Colada Green Smoothie - Prep Pack

Servings: 2 per packet
Method of Storage: Freezer

This is what you'll need:

- 1 banana
- 1 c. of each:
- -Coconut milk - unsweetened
- -Fresh baby spinach
- -Fresh pineapple chunks

Optional Ingredients
- 2 t. raw honey
- ¼ c. ice cubes

This is what you'll need for the garnish:
- Pineapple wedges

Instructions for the Container
1. Add all of the fixings into a reusable plastic container or Ziploc.
2. Make at least a week's worth to save time. Store in the freezer.
3. To Prepare: Pull out one packet of goodies and add to the blender. Add the following to each package:
    a. 1 c. unsweetened coconut milk
    b. 2 t. raw honey – optional
    c. ¼ c. cubed ice – optional
    d. Garnish – wedges of pineapple
4. Blend until you reach the desired consistency.

Conclusion

Thank you for making it through to the *Meal Prep Guide: Time Management for the Kitchen*. Let's hope it was informative and provided you with all of the tools you need to achieve your goals - whatever they may be.

The next step is to decide how dedicated you are to the process. You can begin small to see how well you can adjust to the methods used in successful meal preparation. Make a list of the food items which are your favorites and make a shopping list.

You can go big and use a spreadsheet to lay out the weekly or monthly menus. Each of the recipes provides you with the information needed to keep your refrigerator and freezer stocked with tasty snacks and meals whenever you are hungry.

A busy lifestyle doesn't mean you have to be hungry or eat junk food just because you don't have time to prepare a full meal. You have all of the keys to a successful meal plan at your fingers. Dive in, get organized, and enjoy!

Finally, if you found this book useful in any way, a review on Amazon is always appreciated!

Index for the Recipes

Sushi Jar – Deconstructed
Turkey Taco Lunch Bowls

Soups

Apple Butternut Squash Soup
Broccoli Soup
Fresh Tomato Soup
Sweet Potato Peanut Stew

Chapter 5 - Dinners

Apricot- Ginger Chicken
Broccoli Quinoa Bowl for Dinner
Chickpea & Butternut Fajitas
Cilantro Lime Chicken & Cauliflower Rice
Curried Chickpea Bowls
Greek Chicken
Power Bowl Essentials
Quinoa Green Burritos
Ramen Noodle Salad
Roasted Sausage with Vegetables
Southwestern Black Bean Couscous Salad
Tahini Harissa Buddha Bowl
Tofu Burrito Bowl

Soup

Chicken Soup in the Pot
Creamy Vegetable Soup
Mason Jar Pho Soup
Peanut & Sweet Potato Stew
Tortilla & Chickpea Soup

Chapter 6: Lunch Box Specials

Avocado Chickpea Salad Collard Wraps
Ham & Cheese Croissant
Peanut Butter - Banana & Honey Sandwiches
Pesto Chicken Pita Pockets
Stuffed Bagel Sandwiches

Chapter 7: Desserts

Almond Butter - Brown Rice Crispy Treats
Chia Seed & Ginger Grapefruit Pudding
Donuts in a Minute
Gingerbread Granola
Parfaits on the Go
Peanut Butter & Chocolate Baked Oatmeal Cups
Peanut Butter Muffins

Acai Bowls

Grccn Tropical Bowl
Peanut Butter Loco Hawaiian
Rainbow Bowl

Ice Tray Smoothies
Coconut Water & Mixed Berry Smoothie
Mango & Pineapple Yogurt Smoothie

Chilly One-Serving Smoothies
Chocolate Chip Mint Smoothie
Green Tropical Smoothie
Mixed Berry
Strawberries & Chocolate

Other Tasty Smoothies

Banana Strawberry & Green Smoothie
Pina-Colada Green Smoothie - Prep Pack